Acopuncture & +

Self talk - Saying out W d whad is
going on.

benzo.org.ok

1

WORSE THAN HEROIN
The World's Most Difficult Addiction Problem
By E. Robert Mercer

This a true story. The author is one of millions upon millions of people who are, will be, or have been addicted to a classification of drugs know as benzodiazepines (benzos). It is the largest single addiction problem on planet Earth. Benzos are legal. Their effects are ghastly.

If you live in western society, where bioremediation of illness is worshipped, where we teach our children that popping pills will make you well, it is an almost certainty that either you, a family member or friend is taking one or more benzos.

And if you want to help them, pass on a copy of this book. Sometimes fear is an effective motivator.

Dedicated to all the brave people who have fought, are fighting and will yet fight their way to benzo freedom. Also dedicated to my father, who has been a constant source of love in my life.

On the Cover: "The Scream", by Edvard Munch

1ST Edition

ISBN 978-1-4357-1658-8

Table of Contents

NOTE: Any statements made about individuals in this book, including their actions and words, are not statements of fact, but rather represent the opinion of the author.

Introduction

Worse Than Heroin

Most of us have seen the documentaries on television, listened to the human-interest stories on NPR or read accounts about the ravages of heroin addiction. In some cases, our families have been touched by a loved one, hopelessly addicted to this illicit drug. It isn't pretty and it often tears families apart. Tragically, addicts overdose and die all too often. Yet, there is another drug, or class of drugs, the benzodiazepines, that is far worse than heroin. Why? Read on.

1. **Benzodiazepines are <u>legal</u> and widely prescribed by physicians.** Estimates range from 10 – 50 million unique prescriptions in a year. They are prescribed for reasons ranging from muscle cramps to coughs to anxiety to seizures. They are prescribed far beyond the recommended time frame as a matter of course. *Benzodiazepine addiction is the largest addiction problem in the world.*

2. **Benzos are highly addictive with potentially fatal consequences.** Let's stop saying that we might develop a "dependence" on them. Let's tell it using words that more *accurately describe the danger.* They are addictive, plain and simple. Dr. Heather Ashton, likely the world's foremost authority on benzodiazepines states that the individual who uses benzodiazepines for 6 months has a 50% probability of addiction. After one year of use, the number jumps to nearly 100%!

    Until the time comes that we systemically refer to this as benzodiazepine *addiction,* as opposed to *dependence,* we will never even begin to convince our government or medical community to deal with this problem properly. Let's stop using words that *sound more benign* to describe the problem.

Further, as opposed to accidental overdoses experienced in heroin detox, some benzodiazepine sufferers, while a distinct minority, find no way out of suffering and commit suicide. Suffering and suicide; this is serious business.

3. **The vast number of symptoms in benzodiazepine addiction is staggering.** Many people who try to withdraw from benzodiazepines experience 20, 30, 40, or even 50 or more symptoms, many of which are brutal all by themselves.

4. **Benzodiazepine withdrawal lasts well beyond the typical 1–2 week detox that heroin addicts suffer through.** Once addicted, attempts to withdraw are often nothing short of a horrific, daily battle against symptoms that may last for months and even years, well past the last dose. According to heroin addicts themselves, withdrawal from this class of drugs *makes heroin detox look like a "walk in the park"*. It is fairly common practice for heroin addicts to use the tranquillizing effects of benzos to mitigate the "high" associated with their drug use. Therefore, this is a group of individuals who have experienced both benzodiazepine addiction and withdrawal as well as heroin addiction and detox. They know which one is worse.

5. **Benzodiazepines can produce permanent damage**. Dr. Heather Ashton, widely regarded as the world's preeminent expert on benzodiazepine addiction, has recently published papers that indicate permanent brain damage is possible in 15 – 25% of those who become addicted.

6. **Commonly accepted protocol about how to withdraw once someone is addicted is outdated, in some cases nothing short of cruel, and severely increases the probability of protracted withdrawal.** The medical community as a whole in the U.S. has not yet latched on to what is clearly the safest and best method known, the Ashton

slow taper. The currently accepted inpatient model can only be described as brutal, a "cold-turkey" stoppage with Phenobarbital to stop seizures.

As you read this book, please remember that it is the story of one strong-willed person, not a criminal, with no psychiatric history of any kind, a non-smoker and non-drinker, who found himself addicted to a benzodiazepine, a legal drug. Remember, too, that there are many others who are in full knowledge of this enemy and who are at this very moment fighting the fight of their lives, waging a battle against this legal addiction. There are likely millions more who are symptomatic in some way and do *not* know what is wrong with them, and still millions who are essentially a ticking time bomb, as it is just a matter of time before their addiction surfaces. The truth is that a few of them will get lucky and never become addicted. And it seems that about half of those who become addicted can escape withdrawal symptoms if they withdraw properly. No one, as yet, understands why this is so. On the other hand, sometimes severe withdrawal symptoms present after very short-term use (weeks) and can persist for a long period of time.

Remember, too, that the author's experience is likely the median experience. In other words, it is my opinion that about half of those who find themselves caught in the clutches of this addiction with bizarre, unrelenting, ever-changing symptoms will have a more difficult experience, and about half will find a kinder path to varying degrees. This book is the story of one man's journey through two difficult periods, back to back: first Post Traumatic Stress Disorder treated with benzodiazepines, and then Benzodiazepine Addiction and Withdrawal. The lesson is simple. Do everything humanly possible to avoid these ghastly drugs.

*They are **worse than heroin.***

8

*He was like a seed buried too deep in the soil to which the light
had never penetrated, and which, therefore, has never forced its
way upward to the open air, never experienced the resurrection of
the dead. But seeds will grow ages after they have fallen into the
earth; and indeed, with many kinds, and within some limits, the
older the seed before it germinates, the more plentiful the fruit.
And may it not be believed of many human beings, that, the great
Husbandman having sown them like seeds in the soil of human
affairs, there they lie buried a life long; and only after the upturning
of the soil by death, reach a position in which the awakening of their
aspiration and the consequent growth become possible. Surely He
has made nothing in vain.*

- George Macdonald, "The Wind from the Stars"

Chapter One: Detour

On the morning of Friday, Oct 25, 2002, I had no idea that the
world as I had known it would come crashing down, only to be
ultimately replaced first by Post Traumatic Stress Disorder, and then
by something far worse: the bizarre, unforgiving, relentless world of
benzodiazepine addiction and withdrawal. I did not know that I was
on the edge of a 2-year journey into a place so dark and so horrific
that I would consider something that was completely antithetic to
my nature in 50 years of earthly existence: suicide. Now, over three
years later, I am well again, unlike many benzo sufferers whose
journey has been, unbelievably worse, *sometimes far worse*, than
mine.

In this book, I will focus most of my energy on my
benzodiazepine journey, though certainly PTSD was no picnic.

Some who find themselves face-to-face with benzodiazepine withdrawal, while a distinct minority, do not survive, unable to face the seemingly unending, daily battering anymore. The only future they know is filled with ever-changing, unyielding suffering. There is no way out but to die.

If, through the Grace of God, sheer luck or some combination of the two, someone in benzodiazepine withdrawal manages to discover what is actually wrong with them, their future is still uncertain. At this point in time, they are faced with general medical ignorance so pervasive that it is quite possible they will find themselves with a physician who is unaware even of the existence of benzodiazepine addiction. Then, the benzodiazepine withdrawal sufferer, who has likely discovered the truth from the Internet, has a real challenge: guide the physician through a crossover and tapering process that will take anywhere from a few months to a few years. All the while, the benzodiazepine addict is in horrific withdrawal, living on the edge of the hope/fear dichotomy that a perhaps skeptical physician will pull out of the process. If that happens, the benzodiazepine withdrawal sufferer, without Valium (the proper benzo version to withdraw from), must find an open-minded, knowledgeable physician, or they face the possibility of seizures and death (at the higher doses) if they are forced to suddenly stop the drug.

On the other hand, if no physician in the victim's world will accept the self-diagnosis and then jump on board with the proper protocol, the benzo sufferer has no choice but to attempt to taper off their form of benzodiazepine (that which has been prescribed by their doctor likely years ago) on their own, an extremely difficult, almost impossible and sometimes intolerable task. This is called a direct taper. Once addicted, the vast majority of direct tapers fail, ultimately resulting in reinstatement. Additionally, with each reinstatement, future attempts at tapering become more difficult. Xanax is one of the most difficult to withdraw from directly, and it is now the most widely prescribed benzodiazepine.

Tragically, at this point in time, most people who do not know what is wrong with them never find out. They simply push deeper

Then Klonpin (its equ

11

and deeper into the world of benzo withdrawal symptoms, which is not unlike a trip into the Twilight Zone. Simply put, they can reach a point where reality is not the same anymore as they wait for symptoms to overwhelm their existence. I shudder to think what an attempt at recovery would be like for them. I was on Lorazepam, a generic form of Ativan, for "only" 8 months or so, tapered off far too quickly (about 3 weeks), only to discover my addiction and be forced by brutal symptoms into reinstatement. Having said that, it appears that there isn't a linear relationship between length of time on a benzo and length of withdrawal after addiction occurs. While there is likely a positive correlation, there are many exceptions. I have seen some individuals take 6 – 12 months to taper off their benzo after a relatively short duration of usage (4 –6 weeks) and a relatively low dosage. Some of these people continue to have symptoms well beyond "the last bit", and sometimes these symptoms persist for years.

Further, those who are fortunate enough to have a physician who recognizes the symptoms for what they are, an addiction to a prescription medication, often find themselves subjected to mainstream medicine's approach to solving the problem: stop the drugs cold-turkey and take Phenobarbital to ward off seizures (in-patient approach) or taper down far too quickly, thereby risking seizures and death (outpatient approach). The risk of seizures is far more likely at high dose stoppages. And if they make it past that, their symptoms are severe beyond description and their journey to recovery may well take years of brutal suffering. And very importantly, any withdrawal technique other than the crossover and slow taper, described in detail in this book, dramatically increases the risk of protracted withdrawal, which essentially means that no one knows how long the suffering will last.

There is a better way, yet it is only slowly being recognized by physicians as the safest, most successful approach. Why? Because the single largest source of physician education about prescription drugs in this country is, believe it or not, pharmaceutical drug representatives, men and women who appear at medical practices, solely intent on selling their wares. They come armed with computer printouts of every prescription that every doctor in that practice has written. They make suggestions about new medications, and sometimes offer incentives to doctors so that they will then prescribe them more often. No medical practice is immune from these visits, which happen at a stunningly high frequency, multiple times a day. They are not bad people. They just don't know about the dark side of medications.

Do not expect these reps to walk into a doctor's office and inform them of the dangers of medications. Do not expect them to warn doctors away from using benzodiazepines for more than 4 weeks. That's not how it works. They want to make money. And all the new drugs that reach the market are expensive initially, so naturally reps want high usage. They make more money this way.

And frankly, I don't think it is reasonable to expect every physician in this country to research every new drug. No way. There just isn't time in the life of a doctor to do this. And even if somehow this were possible, do you think that the research on every new drug is completed in an honest manner? Sorry, that's not how it works. Money is the driving force all too often.

So it seems that right now, the only way to educate physicians and the greater medical community about benzodiazepines is for the countless people like me to tell our story.

My own journey would become part of a larger journey, that of a band of worldwide sufferers who somehow managed to be guided to the very same website as I had been. With thousands of members, Benzo.org.uk became known as the best, most comprehensive website on benzodiazepine addiction, withdrawal and recovery in the world, all based on the efforts of one man from the UK, Ray Nimmo. Ray and his league of helpers, know as site administrators and moderators, have saved countless lives, including mine. They have done this quietly, steadily and heroically over many years with no recognition, living in the anonymous, mysterious world of benzodiazepine addiction. Ray's original forum, one aspect of benzo.org.uk, has experienced several iterations, and most of the original volunteer staff have moved on in their lives, replaced by still more wonderful volunteers. This addiction is the largest

Murder or torture!

addiction on the planet, with literally millions of addicts, and as I have already indicated, most do not even know it, *yet*. No addiction on earth is more difficult. And again, I remind the reader that heroin addicts say detox from heroin is *easy* compared to benzo withdrawal.

Government is helpless and even complicit, so inexorably tied to the corrupt side of our large pharmaceutical companies that there seems to be no tangible process by which they can be separated other than through public knowledge. Perhaps this book will help. Countless lawsuits have failed to even get to trial. These pharmaceutical companies, while they do some good in the world, are also guilty of murder and torture. When you begin to develop an understanding of benzo withdrawal, you will come to understand this.

While a few do not survive the attempt to get off these drugs, most just suffer beyond understanding. There are two main reasons for this. First, the sheer number and variety of symptoms is astounding and literally defies rational belief. Second, the path to drug freedom can only come safely through a series of tiny steps that leaves the addict wondering if freedom will ever come. Day after day, week after week, month after month and frequently year after year, the suffering continues, changes, and even gets worse when it seems impossible to do so. But, with superhuman strength and determination, and a great deal of guidance, one can prevail over these poisons. I know this, because somehow, I did.

Out of compassion and moral obligation, I must offer a grim but real warning to millions of Americans (and others): If you *are* taking any one of the following "medications", you are sitting on the edge of a precipice so strange and foreboding, so unremitting and pervasive, so frightening and powerful that not even the strongest amongst you will be able to avoid crumbling, to some extent, under its weight.

Benzodiazepines: Generic (Name brand)
Alprazolam (Xanax)

Bromazepam (Lexotan, Lexomil)
Chlordiazepoxide (Librium)
Clobazam (Frisium)
Clonazepam (Klonopin, Rivotril)
Clorazepate (Tranxene)
Diazepam (Valium)
Estazolam (ProSom)
Flunitrazepam (Rohypnol)
Flurazepam (Dalmane)
Halazepam (Paxipam)
Ketazolam (Anxon)
Loprazolam (Dormonoct)
Lorazepam (Ativan)
Lormetazepam (Noctamid)
Medazepam (Nobrium)
Nitrazepam (Mogadon)
Nordazepam (Nordaz, Calmday)
Oxazepam (Serax, Serenid, Serepax)
Prazepam (Centrax)
Quazepam (Doral)
Temazepam (Restoril, Normison, Euhypnos)
Triazolam (Halcion)

Non-benzodiazepines with similar effects
Zaleplon (Sonata)
Zolpidem (Ambien, Stilnoct)
Zopiclone (Zimovane, Imovane)
Eszopiclone (Lunesta)

If you are not taking these medications, do everything in your power to avoid them, save for the very, very short term (maximum of 2 – 4 weeks) if, as a last resort, you should have no other option. Versed, for example, is used appropriately as a surgical anesthesia and has an extremely short half-life (hours). Benzo addicts, however, should NOT use this drug, especially while in withdrawal.

To understand benzo withdrawal, you must be able to use a little imagination, for the depth of this experience is difficult to express with language. It is my hope, that after reading this book and perhaps others in the suggested reading section on pages 199-200 of this book, you will be a richer being, capable of understanding invisible sufferings such as those associated with benzodiazepine withdrawal. Indeed, awareness of and empathy towards others are two of the many gifts I have been given as a result of my benzo journey. I also hope that you will be mad as hell at the powers that be, as they continue to contribute to the agony known as benzodiazepine addiction and withdrawal. It is my hope, as well, that you either properly get off any benzo you might be on, or, if you are not taking benzos, steadfastly refuse any such prescription except under short-term considerations, again, 2 – 4 weeks.

Invisible

*We must be willing to let go of the life we
have planned so as to have the life that is
waiting for us.*

-- E. M. Forster

Chapter 2: PTSD: A Trip to Hell

Perhaps if I had known more about the nature of stress
breakdowns, I would have been able to glimpse the near future
peering back at me, winking and smiling, waiting to pounce like a
cat on its prey. Perhaps if I had been more self-absorbed, I'd have
been able to step inside myself long enough to see the signs of
impending darkness and the unknown. But fates such as these do
not generally present themselves freely until you are firmly in their
grasp. It is their nature.

My entry into the world of benzodiazepine addiction and
withdrawal was the result of an unfortunate tendency of mine, a
tendency that has been subsequently modified somewhat. It seems
that I spent a great deal of time and energy in trying to manage the
universe. People such as I do that. We care about the underdog, we
try hard to protect others, we have great interest in the health of the
planet, we shudder when we learn of corruption in politics and we
feel helpless in the face of needless death and suffering. So,
whenever we can, in our own tidy little universe, we try to fix
things. We learn how to barter and compromise. We learn how to
negotiate, albeit poorly sometimes, with bad people, often dropping
our left in trust (a boxing analogy), leaving ourselves open to the
quick and deadly right cross. No one can manage the universe, and
while I still maintain a similar worldview as I did in the past, I have
resigned as general manager of the universe. I only work on the
solar system these days, and I keep my left up.

my little corner,

And so it was for me, a 16-year veteran teacher and mid-level administrator at an elementary school in the Northwest. This was the beginning of my entry first into Post Traumatic Stress Disorder and then Benzodiazepine Addiction. At 45 years of age, I was still an idealist in many ways. I believed that, in the face of wrong, one man could speak up loud enough and long enough to make a difference. I believed that doing good, being honest and fair and standing up for what was right was not a choice, rather just the way it was supposed to be. I didn't know about such things as social sociopaths and serial bullies. After all, how could I be bullied? At 6'3" and 280 pounds, who would be silly enough to bully me? I did not realize that in the professional world of education, where I expected everyone to act with fairness and decorum, sociopaths exist.

My simple view of bullying was about to be torn to shreds. There are, it seems, people who spend inordinate periods of time thinking and scheming about ways to expand their own power at the expense of others. And when these people are in leadership positions, they are very dangerous. Until I met Andrew, a serial bully in my humble opinion, I didn't know these people actually existed.

My school had hired a new principal a few years earlier, and I was one of his assistant principals. I had voted against his appointment, had issued a fair warning for what to me seemed like an obvious decision, but was in a distinct minority. During his initial tour of our building with me, he boldly and brazenly directed a strong criticism of the then sitting principal, who was widely revered. I was shocked. If he could resort to this manner of unprofessionalism during the interview process, then what could be expected down the road? The first few years of his tenure had been relatively uneventful, except for the general view, shared by me, that he treated people quite badly sometimes. However, there was a new dynamic emerging. Increasingly, he was turning people against each other, through lies and innuendo. Why? Perhaps a web search for "serial bully" and "sociopath" will help. The short answer: just because, a genetic predisposition to seek chaos amongst people.

Faculty against faculty, parent against parent; with each passing month, it was getting worse. Finally, after observing too many good teachers quit and move on, I had enough. The school I loved had changed and was still in flux. The nurturing environment that I so loved was under attack, both overtly and behind closed doors. At the time, I didn't realize that all the strong personalities were leaving, and that this was not an accident. Andrew wanted them gone, as this would make it easier for him to rule in his Kingdom and easier to have dominion over his subjects.

One fine spring day, I tendered my resignation as an assistant principal, content to proceed with a full teaching load. I was trying to get someone's attention, anyone's attention on the Board, that is. This was, however, the beginning of the end and would lead to my fall (pun intended) on a windy autumn day 18 months later. The behind-the-scenes assassination would soon begin, and any attempt to assert my position would be futile. I should have known something was amiss when not one board member asked me why I had resigned. I subsequently learned that, while I cited differences in philosophy and style as the reason for my resignation (in writing), Andrew simply lied to the Board and made my resignation look completely benign. Regardless, I thought I was hard and enduring bedrock, completely resistant to weathering. I thought I could keep up the good fight indefinitely. How wrong I was.

Of course, it didn't exactly help when, a few months earlier, I supported a colleague of mine in a dispute over a cheating incident. Our one-year replacement Spanish teacher caught a student with his book open, hidden on his lap under the desk, during a test. It was open to the very same page that the testing was covering. It was *possible* that the student was reviewing the material before the test began 20 minutes earlier and just forgot to close it on his lap, and accidentally found himself looking down at it without realizing it was open. Small possibility. But, no matter, the protocol for this matter was clear. The student was found with the book open during the test. The student must receive a zero. The teacher appropriately came to me, an assistant principal, for advice. It seemed clear, a typical case. But then the new teacher, obviously distraught,

announced the kicker. The student was Andrew's seventh-grade
son. Gulp. The teacher had clearly been informed by colleagues
about Andrew's potential. I supported the teacher 100%, even
though I was subjected to a relentless battering on Andrew's part to
convince me that his son was not cheating and to remove the zero.
This went on for about 2 weeks, nearly daily. I'd get called to his
office about some small matter and then the conversation would
inevitably turn to his son and the incident. He even asked me
directly if I believed his son, who claimed to be an innocent victim.
I properly responded that my individual belief was irrelevant, that it
was inappropriate to ask me this, and that I had followed the
protocol correctly. He continued pressing, and I continued to say
the same thing. How utterly inappropriate it was for him to do this,
using his position in an attempt to exert power over me in favor of
his own son. As always, I maintained the composure of the
consummate professional. Translation; I kept my cool. Looking
back, I should have gone to the Board with this immediately. But
that would have been scary, as it could have resulted in my
termination.

Ultimately, I became the chair of a small group of faculty that
were elected to represent the faculty. I pushed the envelope, seeking
a grievance procedure (fully authorized by a faculty vote) in the
event of unethical behavior on the part of any principal, present or
future, directed at a faculty member. When I published a draft
version, all hell broke loose, and I was targeted as "the trouble
maker". While I suspected that the boss would be unhappy, I
underestimated the ferocity of the attack. Mostly I was simply
trying to do good, to protect in some small way those who would
come after me, since I thought I might soon leave by choice anyway.
Why not leave a legacy of fairness behind? Why not do the right
thing?

A barrage of memos was exchanged. A giant split emerged
within the faculty, with about half in full support of me, and the
other half either supporting Andrew or being fearful of what would
happen if they openly supported me. All along, I kept thinking that
any day Andrew would ultimately understand that I was just seeking

serial bullies .

an honest, open way of dealing with conflict. Simply put, this was naïve and foolish on my part. Knowing what I know now about serial bullies, all of my attempts at fairness were more likely perceived by Andrew as signs of weakness and opportunities to destroy me. Then, after a huge attack on me and my committee colleagues at a faculty meeting and his subsequent repeated refusal to talk about the attack (four requests for meetings were simply denied), there was a period of relative calm. Days went by with silence and an air of professionalism. During this calm, an attack was being planned. I did not comprehend four main points at the time.

1. I was feeling a tremendous amount of responsibility to the faculty who had duly elected me as their representative. I had been considered to be one of the pillars of this faculty. I felt strongly that they were depending on me to do the right thing. I believed I was doing the right thing for the good of the many, and to this day, I still believe it. I couldn't let them down.

2. I underestimated the effect of this weight of responsibility in a heavily conflicted, contentious environment. I did not realize the toll it was taking on me. It was essentially a 2-year battle at the time, with ever-increasing contentiousness.

3. Andrew was way ahead of me, having lied to the full board of trustees and some faculty about the reason for my resignation, presenting a completely benign untruth, and lying about my intentions and about things I had allegedly done and said. The board had heard about the growing storm from only his side, since faculty members were forbidden to speak to board members about meaningful work matters. Additionally, the three previous principals had very short tenures and perhaps this board was so loathe to consider another, that it simply stopped caring in order to make their lives easier and dispel the image of a difficult working environment.

bullies lie

21

4. There was, within me, a lingering residual stress from a divorce 2 years earlier and the enveloping stress that had been part of my life prior to that.

And so there I was, ripe for the picking, laden with stress and the weight of responsibility to others. Then, after that brief period of calm and composure, I received a memo asking me to meet with Andrew and Tom, who was the President of the Board. I was, as always, hoping for the best. Maybe Tom had prevailed upon Andrew to do the right thing. After all, the grievance process that I had drafted was overly fair and actually left any final decision with Andrew himself.

I had agreed with my 2 committee colleagues that I would not discuss the substance of the main issue without one of them being there. I was prepared to listen to reason and be open-minded about any counter suggestions.

Yet, inside, I was as fragile as I had ever been in my life, an egg ready to crack, a jigsaw puzzle ready to be taken from its finished form and scattered about.

As you journey through life, take a minute every now and then give a thought for the other fellow. He could be plotting something.

-Hagar the Horrible

Chapter 3 : The Attack

When I sat down that Friday morning in Andrew's office, I was still hopeful. Hope vanished in seconds; the meeting began with a bang. Two adults, one my immediate supervisor and the other the President of the Board, were both actually yelling at me, accusing me of causing trouble and being a malcontent in general. I was to blame for all the unrest. My brain was not prepared for this. It was a shock. Yelling from 2 different places. Fingers being wagged at me, lies, falsehoods, exaggerations, and angry faces were right in front of me, in a closed room. I started taking notes and Tom yelled at me about that and suggested it was just another example of my trouble-making. Soon enough, my hands started shaking and I became unable to write legibly. I tried to hide that, but it was almost impossible. I pressed my two hands hard onto my note pad, one hand holding the back of the pad and the other pressing in with the pen and heel of my hand. My hands and feet were suddenly freezing. I believed was dealing with despicable creatures, but all I could do was muster a few angry questions to Andrew; his answers were complete, utter lies.

At one point, about 30 minutes into the meeting, Tom became worried, apparently having noticed that my demeanor was odd, that something was wrong. He asked me, "Why are you glaring at me?" I said sternly, "Because I want you to get it!". My mouth was as dry as it had ever been. My hands were shaking. My speech patterns were beginning to change towards the end of the meeting, and I had trouble being coherent, with stuttering setting in.

I left the meeting abruptly and forcefully, throwing open the door with a crash. I was trembling and couldn't stop. My sentence structure was slowly departing. I would begin a thought, stop, insert another, stop, attempt to finish somehow, and it was getting steadily worse. I was trying my hardest to regain my composure. It wasn't working. I noticed people, students and faculty/staff, looking at me with concern. They had never seen me like this. Indeed, I had never *been* like this.

By the afternoon, one of my colleagues, Dana, was in my classroom expressing concern about me. She sent my incoming science class back to their 5th grade homeroom teacher. She kept me isolated from the school for the rest of the academic day. To this day, she is a dear friend. I didn't know it then, but one of the students went back to that classroom and said, "I think Mr. Mueller is having a breakdown".

But I had made a commitment to coach a lacrosse game after school for a colleague. My symptoms receded a bit as I forced my thoughts to the game and my obligation to honor my commitment. I called my wife, Maddie, and told her that she should come a little early to the game, since I wasn't feeling right. I told her the meeting was awful, the worst of all the possible scenarios, beyond the worst I had imagined. I knew she could tell something strange was happening, but she tried not to let on.

During the game, I was freezing. I worked hard to keep my thoughts away from the confusing meeting earlier in the day. Andrew was there, I suppose to keep an eye on me given my odd behavior. I did not look at him. I wanted to punch him. He was, in my humble opinion, a liar. As the game drew to a close, I began feeling worse again. A parent spoke to me for a few minutes about soccer, but all I could do was offer small, short answers. I do not know if they made any sense.

By the time I got home, I was stammering. I couldn't explain myself well, but I knew I wasn't myself. I had no clue what had hit me. I couldn't explain it well, but something I had never experienced called clinical anxiety was slowly but steadily creeping into my life. I had no idea it would be an almost constant companion for nearly 2 years. I had no idea that I was in the process of suffering a psychiatric injury called Complex Post Traumatic Stress Disorder.

Windy Evening

This old world needs propping up
When it gets this cold and windy.
The cleverly painted sets,
Oh, they're shaking badly!
They're about to come down.

There'll be nothing but infinite space then.
The silence supreme. Almighty silence.
Egyptian sky. Stars like torches
Of grave robbers entering the crypts of the kings.
Even the wind pausing, waiting to see.

Better grab hold of that tree, Lucille.
Its shape crazed, terror-stricken.
I'll hold the barn.
The chickens in it uneasy.
Smart chickens, rickety world.

-   *Charles Simic*

Chapter 4:   Teetering

Note: A significant portion of my memory of the next 7-8 months is missing. I have compiled a good portion of the chapters that apply to this time frame, varying in quantity from chapter to chapter, from the recollections of friends and family in conjunction with my own recollection. The timing of actual events may well be slightly different.

Evening found me alternately sitting in a high back chair in our dining area, standing up suddenly, pacing around the kitchen and then back to the chair. Restless is an understatement. My stomach wasn't right. It felt like something awful was about to happen. Inside my head, unknown to anyone, a series of intrusive replays was in its infancy, and a new sort of self-talk was also being born. Ultimately during the next two years, this self-talk would be my most powerful weapon for survival.

> *That "meeting", that freaking "meeting" is making me upset. That wasn't a meeting. More like an orchestrated attack. Yelling at me, wagging their goddamn index fingers at me. I should have grabbed those grubby little fingers and bent them back until they apologized. ANDREW was the problem and he had managed to convince Tom and other board members that it was ME. I knew many of those people. I taught their goddamn kids. What the hell was wrong with them? Are they stupid? Okay, Okay. Calm down, Sam. Relax. Just breathe slowly and deeply. What should I do? How do I get these people to recognize that they were victims, too? Yes, that's it. They were victims, too. Okay, now what. Wait. The letter. The letter! THE LETTER! YEEEESSSS!*

Thinking of the letter helped me, gave me hope again. The day before the meeting, in a fit of preparation that defied my foolish tendency to hope for the best, I managed to write a letter to the Board of Trustees. I wasn't certain that I would ever use it, but I wanted to be prepared. There was a Board meeting approaching. It was a simple, short request for a meeting, based on my now 18-year tenure at the school, my 8 years as an Assistant Principal, and my position as Chair of the Faculty Committee. The letter identified my concerns. Included in the list of concerns was a statement that indicated I felt that Andrew had slandered me in the last faculty meeting. I also wanted the opportunity to state my case as to why this man was hurting the school I loved. I wanted to talk about all the good teachers who had left. I wanted to talk about all the lies and the information that had been withheld from them. I wanted them to know how unhappy a place our school was becoming. Yes, I still had hope. I asked my friend Dana to mail those letters on Friday afternoon. Perhaps I managed to mail them myself; I am not certain. My symptoms seemed to ease a bit again as I focused my energy on those letters and hope.

As I fell off to sleep, short-lived images of the meeting flashed through my head. Visuals, different than a dream. More like a still shots from a camera, fading in and out. Flashes of faces. Oh Lord, this was but a little tidbit, a small taste of the future, a future that I could not yet comprehend.

I am up early the next day.

Maddie calls the doctor. No appointment. But she calls anyway. Says it is an emergency. I am anxious, edgy, and short breaths prevail. My stomach is churning and churning. Strange feeling there. (Memory of the letter is temporarily gone.) We're here. This uncomfortable, crappy stomach feeling stinks. I don't like the waiting room. Too many people. Too long a wait. What the hell is going on? That lady was here after me. Why is she going in? I'm going to say something. I tell Maddie. She says it's okay. I trust her. I do not like sitting here. I feel unsettled. I want to go, but I cannot. I need help. Quickly, please. I hate this feeling inside me......what is it? Why can't I just calm down and make it go away?

Maddie is and will become ever so much more, my connection to hope, the only constant in an ever-changing world filled with unknowns.

They call my name. Christ, it's about time. We go in. Maddie tells her what's wrong. My stomach is churning. I have to keep moving. I didn't even know the right word. How do I describe this? It's just that something is wrong.

28

Something really bad. I can't explain it well. What the hell is wrong with me? I don't like the way I feel. Never felt it before. Something feels really wrong. Something is going to happen. The physician's assistant writes this all down. Asks some questions. My thoughts are angry. That was redundant! Jesus! Didn't you hear my answer? Are you deaf? I just answered that!

I answer as best I can, forcing myself to be nice. I feel awful.

THEN SHE ASKS ME IF I CAN GO BACK TO WORK. Tears suddenly well up in my eyes. Fear says hello. I remember this well. My stomach says no. My voice chokes. I say no. SHE ASKS WHY NOT. I search for an answer that makes sense. Nothing does. What do I say? I am afraid to go back. How can I possibly say that? A man my age. My size. Afraid. Maddie tries to explain. I interrupt. Loudly. "I JUST CAN'T!" The Physician's assistant stares at me and says, "Generalized anxiety". They knew me there. Sam isn't like this. Okay, Okay, so there's some words. Good, good, good. Wait a minute. So what. So what? What does it mean? Sounds like a catch-all diagnosis. I remember that word. I worked in a psych hospital. Whenever something isn't clear, it's "generalized". Forget it, Sam. Doesn't matter. It's something. Progress, at least. She's writing me a note. No work. Doctor's orders. Relief. A little, anyway. Thank you God. Thank you lady. Don't have to go back there yet. That place scares the hell out of me.

Remember your humanity and forget the rest.

-Albert Einstein

Chapter 5: Save For a Rainy Day

*Still here. What is she doing? Oh. She's writing
something. A prescription. For anxiety. Not very
much. .5 mg of something. What is it? Lorazepam?
Oh, Lorazepam. Same as Ativan. Generic. Think
I've heard of that. 3 times a day. As needed for
relief of anxiety. Oh good. There's something that
can help me. Can't be too bad for me. But only half
a milligram. Relief. I'd like some of that. Wait a
minute. Only half a milligram. Christ. How can that
help? Half a freaking milligram. TAKE A DEEP
BREATH. It doesn't help. Nothing does. Jesus.
God. I hate this feeling. Why am I thinking so many
bad words? I can't think right, either. Something is
wrong. Something is wrong. What is it! I can't
figure this out. I'm not thinking clearly. Shit! I want
to curse out loud. I want to go to sleep.*

Maybe this Ativan will help me.

In the middle of the journey of our life I came to myself within a dark wood where the straight way was lost.

-Dante Alighieri

Chapter 6: The Disintegrating Man

At home, I can't stop pacing, can't stop the feeling in my upper abdomen. Nothing I do changes it. And I don't seem to be able to control my thoughts as usual. Whenever I force myself to think about something different, within seconds I'm back at that G.D. meeting or back to focusing on the feeling in my stomach.

> *Churning, churning, makes me want to get up and go somewhere, anywhere, outside, around the driveway, over and over. Something has to help, and nothing else is working. This so-called medicine is doing nothing. Squat. Zero. Zilch. Nada. For Christ's sake, how could it? It's only half a milligram. 28 milligrams to an ounce. I think. So that means ……..so that means ………it means something……..I can't quite figure it out …….well, it's really small, so how could it possibly help. WHAT ON EARTH WAS SHE POSSIBLY THINKING? Jesus, what a waste of time. IT DOESN'T HELP. Half a goddamn milligram. What's that? It's next to nothing. I've measured milligrams. They're tiny. Teeny tiny. I've measured them in class. Jesus, I remember ……..there are 28 grams in 1 freaking ounce. How can half of one MILLIgram of them do ANY*

FREAKING GOOD? There's 1000 of them in 1 gram! Is that right? I think so. I do not know right now. Why I can't remember something this simple? What is going on? What is happening to me? Forget it. Forget it! Jesus, it almost hurts to think. Stop it.

Maddie assures me throughout the weekend that the Physician's Assistant was unwilling to prescribe a significant dose because my regular doctor must do that, or because they must find the smallest effective dose. The last part makes the most sense. No need to give extra, unnecessary medicine. I understand this completely, but the bottom line is that I am getting worse.

Saturday night and Sunday night I have only one dream, over and over, still resembling a normal dream state. "The meeting" floats in and out of my sleep, different parts, fingers wagging, angry faces, closed door. In my dreams, I am focused somewhat on getting out of that room. Trying to figure that out. I don't remember thinking that at all during the actual event. But the closed door clearly is a major player in my growing injury, literally or symbolically or both.

Soon, normal dreams would cease, to be replaced by extraordinarily vivid replays of the meeting, over and over, countless times, night after night after night. For weeks into months on end, this is the only "dream" I will have. Very soon, the "dream" will become a video replay of the meeting that is so real, so precise, and so incredibly repetitive that I am able to write a verbatim transcript. It will be like watching a video of the event. No matter how hard I try to get this video out of my head, I can't. It repeats at will, thousands and thousands of times, in dreams and during waking hours. I have absolutely no control over it.

Maddie is as angry as hell. I've never seen her like this. Married to the now disintegrating man for only 2 and ½ years, she has been the model of poise, grace and charm, a loving, nurturing human being. But she is furious. Holy cow, I don't know what to think, besides the obvious. She loves me, someone has made me ill, and something is going to happen. Good.

This has got to stop. How long will it continue? Come on, do something, Sam. Figure it out. You've always been able to problem solve. Get your head together. Focus. What is bloody happening? Got to sleep. Now THAT'S something I can do. Sleep. Only one problem. Even in sleep, I can't shake this. Gotta try, though.

Maddie and I discuss Monday morning. A passing thought that I'll feel better by then jumps into my brain and then disappears quickly. No way. NO WAY. Holy God, no way. Maddie decides to visit Andrew first thing Monday morning. I get pleasure from this, and actually chuckle inside a bit at the thought of what will follow. In days to come, happiness will not exist anywhere in creation. It helps to laugh, even though humor is hard to find right now. Maddie is kind, loving, caring, but there is another side to her. She is quite brilliant, having received a full academic scholarship to an Ivy League university. She does not like conflict, but when fully motivated, she is difficult to debate, possessing extreme clarity of mind and an incredible, nearly photographic memory of conversation. If Andrew says anything stupid or contradictory, Maddie will quickly and adeptly jump on it. In my heart, I know she loves me and will stand tall for me. But I just wish I had been able to do it myself before this happened. Someday, I'll have my chance.

Maddie walks into the school office just after morning arrival and directly, over secretarial protests, into Andrew's office. She yells, "YOU'VE MADE MY HUSBAND SICK!" Everyone hears her. I'm not there, but, as expected, Maddie remembers the entire exchange. The office, filled with people at this time of day, heard the "conversation". I don't really want to think about it too much. But it was good that Andrew was on the defensive for a change. I do feel a tad better emotionally after hearing of this exchange, feeling like somebody finally had the courage to "tell him off". After all, my dear wife was speaking the truth. That's all I ever did, and look where it got me. Doesn't matter. I am who I am.

We went to see my regular doctor, a man who I still deeply trust, and he decided to increase my dosage of Lorazepam to 1 mg, tid. (3 times a day) I was pleased, as he indicated that this drug was very effective in relieving anxiety. When I took the mid-day dose, it did offer *some* relief, a tad, for which I was extremely grateful. The churning in my stomach didn't vanish, but it was more tolerable for a few hours. I continued to wonder how such a low dosage of any medication could be effective in any way. One milligram? Geez, that's miniscule. Maybe, I thought, this was actually a placebo that I was ingesting, and they were just seeing how I would respond. Oh, if only I had been that lucky. I had no clue whatsoever that I was taking into my body one of the most dangerous, addictive drugs on the market, one of the many, many benzodiazepines.

As the day wore on, though, my thoughts went to the letter and the timing. All of the Board members had, by now, received a copy of my letter. Now bear in mind that approximately 16 years earlier, the Board had fully recognized, via a letter from the Board President, the committee that I now chaired, as a separate and distinct committee from the school hierarchy, completely autonomous. The committee by-laws had identified the committee as a vehicle for communication with the Board. So, I was fully authorized by the faculty via vote to communicate with the Board, and the Board as a body had fully recognized the committee and its bylaws as legitimate. Logically and ethically, the Board had an obligation to hear me. I wasn't a new hire. I had been one of the teachers at the core of the school for a long time. I was, again, ever so hopeful.

So on Monday evening, at my request, Maddie called one of the Board members, one whom we thought would be the most fair-minded. I didn't feel competent to articulate any position. No luck. The Board had already convened an Executive Session and they were standing behind the boss 100%. Even after hearing some things that had been withheld from her over the past 2-3 years, she would not relent, choosing to reflect an already chosen position. On what grounds, then, did the Board refuse to speak with me? I cannot say. But in the world of schools, particularly non-public schools, the Board can essentially do just about anything it wants, within legal limits. They can choose to not be bound by any sense of decency. It did not matter that they had violated their own written policy of non-involvement in personnel matters. It did not matter that they had been lied to; they didn't know that then, though they should have.

The good news is that the vast majority of non-public school Boards have both higher standards and better instincts that did this board. (The Board that I work for at this writing is highly ethical.) Mostly members of wealthy families, these particular Board Members were not providing meaningful oversight about anything other than money. In my humble opinion, they just didn't care enough. There were warning signs all around. One year, nearly 40% of the staff resigned. True, some reasons for leaving were unrelated to Andrew. But most were. A faculty committee completed exit interviews. They were given to Tom. He may have never showed them to the full board or the executive committee. Numerous letters were written to the Board president, Tom, from parents. Every one that I saw referenced lying on the part of Andrew. It is likely that Tom never shared them with the full Board, though I cannot say for sure. I resigned as assistant principal, a 16-year, highly rated veteran teacher. Children were sent crying from his office and parents were ridiculed (by Andrew) and even, in my opinion, slandered at faulty meetings. This was a small school community. For a Board member to have been ignorant of all these things or most of them was, in my opinion, clearly a choice.

However, one detail should be noted in fairness to this Board. Many of the board members at that time were parents of current students, parents of graduating 9th graders. Since the vast majority of the students at this school went on to the finest private boarding schools in the country, they all needed that recommendation of the Principal. Perhaps, in their inaction, they were protecting their own interests: their children.

35

I can't tell if a straw ever saved a drowning man, but I know that a mere glance is enough to make despair pause. For in truth we who are creatures of impulse are creatures of despair.

-Joseph Conrad

Chapter 7: Man Overboard

It didn't take long for this to sink in. Looking back, I believe that the refusal of the Board to even engage in conversation was equally as critical as "the meeting" in my developing full-fledged Complex PTSD. Both of these events were traumatic to my brain at the time they occurred. Under normal circumstances, a contentious meeting would have not been an issue beyond the expected upset. Under normal circumstances, a denied request for a meeting would have caused me to be disappointed and discouraged, maybe even somewhat angry. But these circumstances were different. Because of constant, relentless stress that existed during my workday, the regular psychological assaults by Andrew, and stress that carried into my evenings and weekends, an injury to the brain was in process. And now the injury was about to grow roots and establish a home within me. It suddenly felt like a blow to the stomach a second time.

It's over. NO MORE HOPE. They didn't even have the Goddamn decency to talk to me. Not even TALK to me.

Refused to TALK to me. What the F are they afraid of?
Assholes. This is wrong. Wrong, wrong, wrong. Now what
the heck am I going to do? Well, I've got a note for now. I
can't go back yet, that's for sure. That man still scares me.
He lies. He schemes. He is hurtful to children. He's a
mean-spirited creep. How much sick time do I have? What
will I do when that runs out? I DO NOT WANT TO TALK
TO HIM ON THE PHONE. I DO NOT WANT TO SEE HIM.
LOOK WHAT HE HAS DONE TO ME. IF I SEE HIM I
MIGHT EXPLODE ALL OVER HIM. I actually could do
that now. Not ever under normal circumstances, but this
was different. I'm sick. I can't predict my behavior. I could
end up in jail.

   I sit in the red wingback chair again. For some unknown reason,
this chair, MY chair, would help me feel safe. I have tried to
understand this even to this day, but other than it was a large,
comfortable chair that was referred to as MY chair, I cannot fathom
why. Like Archie Bunker, I would allow no one to sit in MY chair,
only I was a little more imposing than Archie.

   This night was different. I did not sleep as well. All my life, I
have been a "sleeper", someone who needs at least 8 hours per
night, sometimes more. I can sleep 8-9 hours every day, easily. But
this night would be a night unlike any previous night of my life.
Perhaps I slept 2-3 hours, on and off. I cannot remember. I do
remember the substance of my dreams, which were changing in
quality with each passing night. This night would find me
reviewing the meeting with slightly more detail and also reviewing
what I imagined the voice on the other end of Maddie's phone call
was saying. I did none of this by choice. Image after image after
image. Angry faces, fingers wagging, faces fading in and out,
repeating. I'd become distressed and wake up, stay awake for a
while, go out to my chair, come back in and repeat the whole thing,
not exactly, but nearly.
   During the next 3-4 weeks, my self-talk changed in quality. It
became more choppy, more fragmented as the injury progressed

steadily. I was worried about my future. I felt frightened. Lost. I could not go back to work, yet I had enormous self-imposed pressure sitting on my shoulders. We were in a new house with a hefty mortgage. The loss of a 70K salary would be huge. How were we going to survive?

Real life pressures were bad enough. But a new, emerging fear and perception was growing rapidly, and it would rock me like nothing else ever had. I had been a teacher for over 18 years now. And before that, portions of my jobs for many years involved teaching components. Teaching was a significant chunk of my persona. Sam = teacher was the equation in my brain. The essence of my very *being* was connected to teaching. Now that the teacher part of the equation was gone, and gone for an as yet undetermined length of time, the Sam part was lost. Who was I? I was not present anymore. I do not think this is a concept that most people can possibly understand. How can I explain it sufficiently? How can those of us, untouched by this invisible enemy, imagine our personality, our definition of self simply evaporated? To understand this, I think one must experience it. But I can tell you in one word how it felt: terrifying. Where was I? Where did I go? Would I ever be me again? Who am I now? I don't like me now. It is not unlike a nightmare. A real, living, breathing nightmare. My very being had changed. I simply did not know what to do.

For the first time in my life, I have no answers; not even bad ones. I am completely lost, wandering about in a body that does not know itself.

My response to all of this was to grasp at the only aspect of the past that was near and clear. I latched on to my dear wife like a drowning swimmer clinging to his rescuer. I could not let go lest I drown. I smothered her. She was real. She was a constant. She was incredibly strong, at least for now. For it wouldn't be long before this living nightmare would find her feet, too, in the gathering quicksand that was setting up all about me.

Over the next 18 months or so, I was completely incapable of being a partner in any sense of the word. I was more like a champion anti-partner, one that steadily saps the strength and

38

vitality of the other. As my fears proliferated in number and intensity, part of the PTSD experience, I became worse than child-like. I could not make any decisions, and I could not take any initiative. On the other hand, I *could* be helpless, argumentative, angry and dependent. I *could* sit and stare well. I *could* complain well and say no to any request. I *could* articulate fears poorly but frequently. I *could* repeat myself incessantly, almost to the point of being pure, unfettered babble. I was quite good at annoying others. I became the biggest load anyone else could ever have to carry. No, it was worse. I made Maddie's life truly miserable. Truly.

And then in the late summer and early fall, as PTSD's sun was beginning to set behind the changing hills, it would all fall apart again, with two major differences. It would be far, far, worse, and for about 3 months, no one could ascertain what was wrong. In the end, as the result of dogged determination and some luck, I was able to successfully self-diagnose: benzodiazepine addiction.

Vile deeds like poison weeds bloom well in prison air, it is only what is good in man, that wastes and withers there.

-Oscar Wilde

Chapter 8: Full Bloom

By December, I was in bad shape. I was officially terminated from my position in early December, even though I felt like I had simply "not gone back" and never would. I did not know who I was and that was terrifying. I was not dreaming anymore, thanks to the effects of Lorazepam. I wish it actually had been able to inhibit the constant intrusive replays, both during sleep and wakefulness, replays of that final meeting. It was supposed to do that, I think. It did not. My brain replayed that meeting over and over and over and over. All day, every day. All night, every night. No wonder I was able to make a verbatim transcript. I had the entire bloody meeting memorized, word for word. Now, 4 years later, most of the meeting is completely gone from my memory.

My dosage had been increased again to counteract these replays and other symptoms. I was now taking 2 mg. of Lorazepam (Ativan) tid., PLUS 2 mg. of Clonazepam (Klonopin) before bedtime (some nights, when I felt particularly disturbed by intrusive thoughts). I was sleeping, sleeping, sleeping, but with no standard dreaming. This was not truly restorative sleep. Nothing but replays.

Even while awake, when I wasn't distracted by somebody or something, I would see the exact same replay after replay, over and over, as though there were a video machine in my head.

February found a rumbling in my ears and my head every night that would come and go, several times. I had worn a hearing aid in my right ear for a couple of years or so, but suddenly found that it made me uncomfortable. I remarked several times to Maddie that the hearing in my right ear was diminishing. Even so, the hearing aid only amplified my startle reflex, a remarkable phenomenon. During all waking moments, I felt like I was in a suspense movie at the climax, when the heroine is slowly, slowly, walking through a dark building waiting for something to jump out at her. If I were to go out into public, I would risk suddenly turning at a sound and lashing out at some poor, unsuspecting individual or bolting. Given my size, strength and surprising speed, the results would be really ugly.

I was still thinking that this medication couldn't be a problem, since the dosage was so low. But here's the catch. I had been duped, along with countless other victims, into believing that 1 and 2 were little numbers. Well, they are, of course, and that is a large part of the problem. Unfortunately, 1 or 2 mg. of the new generation of tranquilizers is NOT small in terms of dosage. Not even close. You see, by the end of the day, at times, I was taking the equivalent of 100 mg. of Valium! That's enough Valium to knock out more than one family of human beings. Normally, 10 mg. will send most people into a drugged sleep. But I was functioning on a daily diet of at least the equivalent of 60-100 mg. of Valium. Ativan, it seems, does not have quite the sedating effects of Valium. In any event, it "sounded" small, only 2 mg. of Ativan three times daily. After all, 6 is a pretty small number, too.

The pharmaceutical companies have all sorts of tricks up their sleeves, and this is one of them. After Valium became unpopular (for good reason: people were becoming addicted), they simply reinvented it, with different names, lower-sounding doses and shorter half-lives. In short, they made Valium more powerful, more treacherous, and more palatable.

So instead of prescribing, for example, an initial dosage of 10 mg. of Valium, human guinea pigs were now gifted with only 1 mg. of Ativan or .5 mg of Klonopin (equivalent amounts). Sounds harmless. The number 10 or 20 or 30 sounds much worse than .5, 1, or 1.5 (Xanax, Klonopin equivalents of Valium).

Furthermore, pharmaceutical company reps convinced doctors that this stuff was really good, since it was eliminated from the body much more quickly that Valium. Indeed, this is true for those potential victims not yet addicted. The half-life of Valium is about 8 days. The half-life of Ativan is about 10 hours. That means, essentially, that Ativan leaves the body quickly: half of it in 10 hours, another half in 10 more hours, etc. Good news, right? Yes, if used properly, for no more than 2-4 weeks maximum (and in some cases, even this is too long). But not if the patient becomes addicted, which is far more common than believed by many in the medical profession. In fact, if the patient becomes addicted as I did, the decreased half-life makes things far, far worse, and can, depending on the specific benzo that is being ingested and the individual's ability to metabolize it, produce something called *interdose withdrawal*. This means that the body is screaming out with withdrawal symptoms before the next scheduled administration of the drug.

Before my dreams disappeared completely, I had a sequence of dreams over a 1-week period that was very revealing. I found myself driving a school bus filled with children. As I drove along, I began to slowly lose control of the bus as we went down a hill. The steering wheel would not respond properly, the brakes would not work right, and ultimately the bus would fly off the road over a cliff. One time the steering wheel became a stick and I didn't know how it worked. Another time the brakes caused the bus to speed up. Every night that I had this dream, I would wake up with a start.

Now in full-blown PTSD, I was presenting with a number of classic PTSD symptoms:

anxiety (ever-present)
hypervigilance (feels like and appears to be paranoia but it is not)

a powerfully exaggerated startle reflex
irritability
angry outbursts
intrusive replays
phobias were setting in
irrational behavior
impaired memory (which would get worse)
inability to do previously simple tasks (poor concentration)
feelings of guilt
extremely low self-esteem
anhedonia (inability to feel joy and pleasure)
an overwhelming feeling of injustice (that HAD to be acted on)

   Two stories illustrate some of these behaviors. During one of my
regular visits to the doctor, I was unable to wait inside, preferring to
pace around the parking lot endlessly, until Maddie called me in. It
was hard to sit still in this setting. During my repeated circular trek
around the parking lot, a gentleman in a car began to stare at me
every time I passed by his car. I was wearing my winter ski hat that
never left my head save for sleep, and a large, heavy winter coat. I
must have been a sight to see, a large, hulking man endlessly
circling the parking lot with a determined gait. I noticed this man
staring at me with each loop, and I started to get annoyed. Each trip
around the lot found me angrier and angrier. He kept staring at me.
I started to boil inside. Finally, I had enough. I briskly walked
straight over to his car window (his eyes widened), motioned for
him to roll it down, got about 6 inches from his face and asked him,
"Do you have a (blanking) problem?" He said, "Nooo…", rather
meekly. Slowly, through clenched teeth and eyes turned to daggers,
I then said, "Well then stop staring at me!" I turned away and
continued my journey as though this was a normal exchange. Upon
my next pass by him, his gaze was fast upon a book. Looking back,
I am on the edge of laughter as I think about that poor man. Imagine
a 6' 3" 280 lb. crazy-acting behemoth approaching you in this
manner. I'd like to apologize to him now! But, at the time, my

anger was completely justified and this poor stranger was completely in the wrong.

The startle reflex was a challenge. If I were in close proximity to the telephone when it rang, I would nearly jump out of my skin. If a family member dropped a piece of silverware, I felt like I would hit the ceiling. If someone came from behind me unannounced, I would turn with a jerk ready to defend myself or run. Any stray sound caused me to jump in varying degrees. This is a common symptom of PTSD and, like the others, it cannot be controlled by rational thought.

In approximately the same time frame somewhere between early January and late February, another incident will provide the reader with a clear look into my frame of mind. It was dark, about 7:00 p.m. For some reason, I decided I had to walk into town, approximately 3 miles away, to get a snack. I was angry about something undetermined. The first part of the walk was on a lonely, country road. It was more than dark. Cloud-covered and cold, the night was as black as I can ever remember it. Under normal circumstances, I would never have taken this little journey. Yet tonight, something gave me courage, and I believe it was profound anger. Frankly, nothing frightened me this night. Sometimes anger overwhelmed fear. I just had to go. As usual, I wore my ski hat, a pullover, knitted hat that I wore all the time, every day, inside the house and outside the house. I only removed this hat to sleep. I do not know why. I also wore a large, heavy winter coat, as it was below freezing, and gloves. I took a flashlight. I started. Just by luck, a car was coming just as soon as my feet hit the macadam. It kept its high beams up, and that really ticked me off. So I turned around, jogged to the barn and found a large stick. Off I went again. I set a demanding pace, as though there was truly an important, almost urgent mission within me. But for my heavy breathing and stick tapping the pavement with each stride, it was quiet. I reached the second part of this madcap trip, taking a left onto a more heavily traveled county road. Cars started passing every minute or two, and I was ready for them. I glared at each oncoming vehicle, waiting to see if it dimmed its headlights. If it did, all was well. If it did not, I

44

shined my flashlight directly at the driver and waved my large walking stick menacingly. I did this for about an hour, the full length of the two-way trip. By the grace of God, no one called the police.

I was also locked in a memory-impaired world. One day, I was traveling in a train to NYC to see my lawyer. I was fearful, but tried not to show it. Naturally, I was in a constant scanning mode, my eyes moving from person to person in an attempt to identify potentially dangerous people. I say "naturally", because this is a natural product of the fear level that exists in PTSD: self-protection. Suddenly, a man who had passed the "potentially bad person" test said hello, called me by my first name and reached out a hand. I stared at him while shaking his hand. I did not know him and did not pretend as though I did. He quickly recognized my confusion and told me who he was: Bill, the husband of a close colleague of mine, a man that I had met and spoken with on numerous occasions. Still, blank. Nothing. To this day, I have no memory of having met him previously. Subsequently, I have come to know him and consider him my friend. His wife, a colleague at my former school, has become a dear friend, who supported me through tough times.

Tis an ill wind that blows no minds.

-Malaclypse the Younger

Chapter 9: The Winds of March

With the arrival of March, my anxiety was diminishing to a point at which I thought I *might* be getting better. The replays were fading, almost gone. The hearing in my right ear was still slowly dropping, but I refused to use my hearing aid; sound had become uncomfortable in an undetermined and an as yet unrecognized way, consciously. My memory was still awful. I could not remember meeting people only days after they visited. I could not do simple multiplication in my head. As a veteran math/science teacher, this was disturbing. Why wasn't my brain working right? Normally, I could multiply two 2-digit numbers in my head with ease. Now, I couldn't manage 9 x 12. My typing was exhibiting nmuerous revresals. On a cetiran level, I did fnid all this fasicntaing. When I tried to back my car up, it was an adventure that found me swerving around like a madman. I could not get the concept of direction correct in reverse.

But March brought another change. The anger and mind-chaos that so consumed me at first was now being replaced by a brand new, previously unknown foe: clinical depression. Sure, I had experienced sadness in my life, but this was vastly different. The world was darkening steadily and with increasing speed.

Shit

Overwhelming despair soon overtook me. Frequently, I walked slowly around my oval driveway, over and over for hours, with tears streaming down my face, and I could not determine why. The tears kept coming. I felt like I could die, though I did not actively think about how this might happen. My heart now understands what life is like for the millions of clinically depressed people in the world. Until you feel the ever-deepening darkness, a darkness that feels like a one-way ticket to utter, total despair, you cannot fathom what it is like to be clinically depressed. It is as though you live in a perpetual, moonless, starless, black night, a night devoid of hope and anything even remotely resembling happiness.

> *As I walk around the driveway endlessly, tears blurring my vision, I see a friend peaking out from behind a sycamore tree. She isn't really trying to hide. She wants me to know that she is near, that I am not alone. She has never come this close before, though I have felt her presence. Someday she will hold me in her arms and take me away. I see her and our eyes lock. I want to go to her, but I cannot. I'm still entrenched in this world. It is not yet time for this change, even though a part of me yearns for her comfort and peacefulness, feelings now alien to me. I continue walking. Soon, she is gone, and I feel alone once again.*

Recognizing that something new was happening, I went to my doctor who did exactly what the "textbook" said to do: prescribe an antidepressant. It seems that tranquilizer use after the onset of PTSD frequently results, in time, with a trip into the dark world of clinical depression. Perhaps if I had instead begun to withdraw from the poison named Ativan, my journey would have been different. I cannot say, as no one knows when benzo addiction begins. In some cases, it takes a firm rooting in a matter of weeks. In still other cases (a small percentage), it never happens, though I suspect that the percentage of non-addiction after years of benzo use is much smaller than believed. After taking benzos for years, a person simply loses track of what it is like to "feel normal". They have been cheated out of a normal existence and likely they are on several drugs, each prescribed to counter symptoms not recognized as benzo addiction. In short, they live on a daily drug cocktail.

Not surprisingly, another drug was added: celexa, an SSRI. This classification of drug acts as a serotonin pump, disallowing serotonin from being absorbed and subsequently eliminated quickly from the body. It essentially floods the brain with serotonin. Low serotonin levels are a symptom of clinical depression. I responded to celexa unusually quickly, within 3-4 days. This sort of response takes place in about 3% of the population. Most of us respond after a longer period of accumulation, in a few weeks. Unfortunately, this drug and its companion drugs play havoc with levels of other things in our brain. There are NO, true, *long-term* studies relative to side effects. Those of us who take these meds are guinea pigs on a grand scale. One thing is for certain: they down-regulate serotonin receptors in the brain. Since there is a huge increase in the amount of serotonin, fewer receptors are needed. So, they die back in number. Alas, no one really knows unequivocally what happens biochemically when a patient stops taking the SSRI (slowly, of course). These brain receptors don't, for sure, suddenly and immediately spring back to life after non-use. So what happens? Most people have a difficult time adjusting to a diminished amount of serotonin. Things aren't what they used to be. Readers wishing for a more thorough understanding of this topic should read Dr. Peter Breggin's book, The Antidepressant Handbook. A psychiatrist himself, Dr. Breggin is now one of the leading experts on psychiatric meds like benzos and SSRIs and is staunchly against their use as it is currently defined. The picture he paints as I see it, isn't pretty. He believes, I think, that all psychiatric drugs have one thing in common: they disable the brain.

Then, the pendulum swung the other way. Unbelievably, within 4 - 6 weeks, I was manic. I could not stop talking. I was happy beyond understanding, though it was not a true happiness. It was more like a frantic existence than anything else. I drove people crazy. When they saw me coming, they dove for cover. From one extreme to the other, I felt like a human yo-yo. I wanted to talk

about everything over and over. Oh, Lord, please slow me down.
My eyes felt like daggers, hyper-focused on everyone and
everything. This was quite a roller-coaster. I went to a gathering of
friends one night at Dana's house. I attended only because I knew
everyone. No strangers. Dana's partner, Shellie, had a parrot, an
African Grey, named "Bobby". Every time Bobby squawked, so did
I. All evening, one squawk and then another! I drove people crazy,
but I hadn't laughed so hard in a long, long, time. What a night!
   One day in May, as Spring opened for business all around me, an
odd symptom surfaced. Ignored at the time as "just one of those
passing things" that we all get and can't explain, it was the first
significant hint at the demon emerging within, the first indication
that I was on the edge of the bizarre, unforgiving world of
benzodiazepine addiction. PTSD would soon pale by comparison to
the icy, relentless grip of this monster.

Shit.

Fewer receptors are needed.
(for me.
Serotonin & Norepinepherin.

All psychiatric Drugs They disable the Brain!

49

We can learn nothing except by going from the known to the unknown.

- Claude Bernard

Chapter 10: The Merry, Merry Month of May

To paraphrase a famous astronomer's quote about the universe, I can tell you that Benzodiazepine withdrawal is not only more brutal that you imagine, it is more brutal than you *can* imagine. Nothing in my earthly experience could possibly have prepared me for what was to come. The seed of benzodiazepine addiction had quietly opened within me, and was now growing beneath the surface, unseen and undisturbed, being nourished every day, three times a day by a tiny circular object smaller than a pea that I would grow to hate beyond belief: a 2-mg. Ativan pill.

This odd day in May found me joining my wife at her place of work, the home of a beautiful, multiply-handicapped, 9 year-old boy. Already, she had cared for him for 7 years. I was manic, but as this was early morning and I was a slow "waker-upper", I was still quiet and not yet particularly annoying. I sat in the living room reclining chair, perfectly ready, willing and able, as always, to fall back into the safe, secure hands of sleep. With no more replays at all, anxiety greatly diminished, fears mostly abated, and a small startle reflex still about here and there, I was almost over my PTSD. I was so very happy, completely unaware that the worst had yet to come.

Maddie is just about ready to bring Kristian out to the special school bus he needs. My eyes have been closed, resting on the edge of sleep. I open them to begin the process of arising from the deep, comfortable reclining chair. Suddenly, I feel disoriented and within seconds the world turns sideways visually. I cannot focus my vision on anything. I feel very warm. Nausea, increasing in intensity with light-speed, causes me to quickly find my way to the bathroom for what seems like the inevitable purge. Only a short trip, I hang onto the wall as I wobble oddly to the entry door. I make it. I drop to my knees and have a brief relationship with the toilet bowl. There are several very intense heaves. A very small amount of new liquid appears in the bowl, the tea I had consumed about an hour earlier. I am perspiring profusely, sweat now dripping from my forehead. The world is not in focus. No matter how hard I try, it is simply all mixed-up. I am really confused about what is happening. Within 2-3 minutes, clarity returns first to vision and then to thought. As quickly as it had hit me, it is gone. Maddie, an Rn., rules out a heart attack. So do I. "What the hell was that?" I ask aloud. "Just one of those things, I guess."

This disorientation, though quite brief, was like no disorientation I had ever experienced. I had been dizzy and I had been light-headed in my life. I had known intoxication from alcohol during much younger college days. None of those experiences were like this. The visual manner in which the world became distorted was simply bizarre. And this was but a shallow glimpse of strange things and suffering to come.

Twice within the next week, I experienced almost identical "attacks", except that they lasted a bit longer each time. Finally, I had enough. I concluded it was time to get off the celexa. I stopped "cold turkey", not a smart thing to do at all. But I was completely convinced it was the celexa, a fairly recent addition to my life, that had caused this weird symptom, and I was simply going to stop

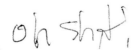

51

taking it. Period. I did not like the feeling I had in these recent "episodes".

It was, of course, in retrospect, the wrong drug to stop. On the other hand, if I had decided to stop the 6-mg. dosage of Ativan cold turkey, I would have risked seizures and even death. As it was, I escaped the stupidity of the sudden stoppage of celexa with no apparent side effects. I was just plain lucky.

At the time I did not know that I had experienced what can only be called *very low-level vertigo*, given the intensity of what I was to experience in the future. Many things can cause vertigo, but not many physicians recognize it as a benzodiazepine addiction symptom. I continued to experience this symptom about once every 2 weeks, still at a very low level until early July. Then it went into hiding, patiently waiting its turn once full-blown benzodiazepine withdrawal was upon me.

*As God and Satan were walking down the street one day,
the Lord bent down and picked something up. He gazed at
it glowing radiantly in his hand. Satan, curious, asked,
"What's that?" "This", answered the Lord, "is Truth."
"Here", replied Satan as he reached for it, "let me have that -
I'll organize it for you."*

- from "Chop Wood, Carry Water"

Chapter 11: Surprise!

Mid-July 2003. I finally have the courage to remove myself from the medication. My doctor, a friend, had allowed me to be in charge of this decision. It was likely because of that friendship and also the understanding that I was generally pretty thorough about investigating meds I had taken, that he did not insist that I get off sooner. But as my psyche had been through the mill, I felt unsafe stopping any sooner. And frankly, there was an almost complete absence of warnings anywhere about the drug I was taking. Yet, I hadn't done a thorough investigation into this drug at all. I was too sick early on. Now, I was ready to begin a new life. I had been hired to teach at a new school, and I was very pleased to have ME back again. I was beginning to plan my classroom and was very excited about it.

My doc had cautioned me to taper slowly off the Ativan, and I assured him I would. Truth is I did not know how slowly I should have gone. But it really didn't matter, because the seed that had quietly germinated within me had been growing stronger and stronger in complete silence, a silence soon to be broken in both a figurative and very literal sense.

I cannot say for sure, but I believe I tapered off the Ativan in about 3 weeks. It may have been less. I don't think it was more than that. Regardless, it was way too fast. However, I felt good about being drug free. Very good. I did not want to take any more medication ever again, if I could help it. Little did I know what the future held.

The hearing in my right ear continued to deteriorate. One day, in close proximity to my day of drug freedom (first round), it was gone. Completely. I was upset. I didn't expect this. Yet, I was dealing with it fairly well. After the audiologist did his thing, the ENT specialist, Dr. Damon, had no clue: a total discrimination loss and an almost total sensory-neural loss. No one had an explanation. I told him about the vertigo symptoms. Maybe it was this or that. Perhaps the medication. But nothing fit right, at least given his knowledge bank.

Now, I officially had a "good side" and a "bad side", just like some of the older people I had known. I was one of them. I could have some fun with this, but I wish it wasn't so.

On Friday, Maddie and I decided to visit a local mountain river stream, runoff from the Cascades, with a waterfall. Though only about an hour away, we had never been there before. It was brutally hot and humid; 97 degrees and high humidity, the manner of day that saps all your strength. At the falls, several people were swimming, and one crazy boy, about 17, jumped into the deep pool at the bottom of the cascading water from the very top of the falls, about 40-feet up. It struck me as both impressive and foolish. We were warned that the water was extremely cold, and the warning was dead on. Man, it was hard to get in, but we both did and had a grand time. Freezing! Argh! It was really fun, more fun than we had together in a long time.

The next morning arrived. About two weeks had passed since I was drug-free, perhaps 10-12 days. I was sleeping in, as usual. Maddie had come in to my bedroom, as we had been sleeping separately since the PTSD had begun, and lay down next to me gently. I felt her presence and smiled. Things were finally getting better, I thought.

I ask her to turn off the alarm. She says it isn't on. I say it is. The radio is on and it is buzzing. Please turn it off. Honey, it's not on, I promise. As I lay there, I suddenly realize that this sound is not external. Panic, almost total, complete panic sets in. I sit bolt upright in the bed, suddenly hyper-awake. My face takes on a pained look. I rub my right ear. There's a sound in it, like a buzzing, metal, generator, jet engine noise. It's not extremely loud, but I can damn well hear it. It's loud enough. I shake my head. I tap my head with my right hand. I put my right index finger in my right ear and move it around and about. I try everything possible.

*Shit! It's not going away. What IS this? Stay calm. It will go away. It has to. I've never heard of this. Maybe I'm dreaming. What is going on? Please be dreaming. A quick please to God that I am. I fail the pinch test. I'm up now, walking quickly to nowhere. Just walking from room to room. Maybe it's a radio in another room. I'm getting scared. I don't know what the hell is happening. **Shit!** ANOTHER thing is happening. What is this? It won't stop! It won't stop! I want it to stop! I can't take much more of this. I hit my head harder. I rub my ear harder and faster. NOTHING WORKS.*

A familiar feeling returns. Anxiety. I thought it was gone, or nearly gone. But here it is again. No, no, no. Please not again.
Maddie has become hopeful that things were getting better, though she is still in energy depletion. I see a stunned look on her face, as if she is about to say, "Please, Sam, no more, no more." But there would be a great deal more.

I have always known
That at last I would
Take this road, but yesterday
I did not know it would be
Today.

        --Ariwara no Narihira

Chapter 12: The Rest of My Life?

 I call my ENT specialist. They have Saturday morning hours, but they have no openings. I tell them it is an emergency and I am coming in anyway, in 5 minutes. I tell them about the sound. By the time I arrive, my logical right-brain thinking has taken over. I am relatively calm. I have sorted it all out in the 3-mile ride in the car.

> *Everything is going to be all right. I'm sure there is an easy answer for this. It's just stupid. How can there be a sound in my head, anyway? I didn't have a head injury. No loud noises. We all get tones in our ears that go away. This was just taking a little longer, that's all. The doctor will know what's wrong. He's a specialist, after all. Maybe it's just a build-up of wax. Yeah, that's it. Or maybe a perforation that is infected. Now THAT'S more likely. I've had a million perforations in my life and gazillions of ear infections.*

 I arrive and announce my presence. I wait about 30 minutes, cool, calm, and collected. Finally, I am called into the examination room. Dr. Lo, one of two partners in this practice and the doctor I have never seen in my previous visits, is very polite and asks many questions. A full, proper smelling out takes place. I feel certain he is on to something. He asks about medications, injuries, and other symptoms. He examines my right ear for a long time. The record reveals to him my total hearing loss. He seemingly reads slowly and carefully. He asks me to describe the sound. He asks when it started. Then he examines my ear again. He takes some deep breaths. He looks at my other ear, the "good" one, even though that has a small hearing loss, too. He reads my record again, only this time he is slowly shaking his head. I don't like that. I'm watching him intently, and now I am getting a little worried. Then he says it. "Tinnitus". I repeat the word. I've heard it. I remember that sometimes elderly people get it. Rock musicians, too. Loud music can cause it. Huh. That doesn't work here.

He explains that in some cases involving a complete loss of hearing, a sort of feedback process can begin. The absence of perceived sound can cause the brain to make up for the absence with this feedback process. I sit and think, quickly, and then ask the logical question. "What can we do?" He suggests that we wait a while to see if it might resolve itself, and that it might well do that. Ah. That does encourage me.

I leave with mixed feelings. I have a name, tinnitus. I have no other answers, but that guy did say it may resolve itself. So I have hope too. When I arrive back home, I explain all this to Maddie. She presents herself as being hopeful and positive, all a good act. She agrees that it will likely go away. The sound, nevertheless, is still there and it is upsetting me. I don't let on. Maddie has been through enough. Jesus, this has been tough on her. I can't let anything else go wrong with me. I've got to figure this out.

The next morning, the sound is gone! Thank you, God! Whew! That had me worried a bit. Okay, more than a bit. I am nearly euphoric about this development, and it reminds me of how I behaved when I was manic. So I exerted just a little control over my "heightened relief". I think of the line in the Wizard of Oz, when Dorothy says, "People come and go so quickly around here!" Instead of people, I have symptoms that do that.

I go to sleep that night with no worries. At some point, I wake up to use the bathroom, as always.

It's back, holy crap, it's back! Shit! And my stomach, that feeling is back!

I take a shower and adjust the spray nozzle to various settings, hoping that its impact on my head will do something. No such luck. I go back to bed, after deciding not to wake Maddie. Why would I do that? She need not know this. I don't want her to know. I have to protect her. By the grace of God, I'm a sleeper. Somehow, I manage to fall off despite the God-awful sound inside my head.

Next morning, Maddie enters my room with her usual, loving manner. "Good morning, Honey. Did you sleep well?" I respond, "Uh-huh". Lousy job, Sam. Didn't fool her at all. She asks what's wrong, and is that sound back again. I acknowledge that it is, but try to play it down. I can't fool her, and she knows I am worried. That same, slightly strained look, almost a grimace, the look that comes with anxiety is on my face again. I cannot hide it and Maddie sees it clearly. We both carry on with the day as best we can.

After a week of on-again, off-again tinnitus, the sound starts to become steadier, almost all the time. It seems louder, too. I wonder if I am going to go mad. What an effective form of torture this could be. Implant something that causes sound inside the head and watch that person go mad. Anxiety is slowly ratcheting up.

*I return at the appointed time to the ENT office. Dr. Damon is there this time. He goes through the same routine as Dr. Lo. Having had some time to piece this together, I ask Dr. Demon, I mean Dr. Damon the question I have been pondering for several days. I have concluded, perhaps out of desperate need to conclude **something**, that the stoppage of the medication is the only logical cause of this. I ask could this possibly be a consequence of stopping the Ativan. He gathers an arrogant, deity-style attitude, scowls and says,* *with a clearly dismissive, drawn out tone, "Noooooo." It was all there in that tone and facial expression. "Who do you, little uneducated man that you are, think you are, daring to suggest something so foolish to me, a d-o-c-t-o-r!" I have never seen this in him before. Good timing in one sense. I am too frightened and upset to let him have it. Any other time, and we would have had a clarification process. Christ. I have almost as much education as he does. And I wasn't an asshole, at least not today. No matter. I buy, however grudgingly, into his D.O.C. model this time. Deity Of Course. He would know. He's the specialist. Specialist. I keep telling myself that this guy is a specialist, so therefore he would know about this sort of thing IN THE EAR. This is his specialty. EAR, Nose and Throat. And it is the first one on the list, too. EAR. It's not third, like THROAT. He should know more about the first thing on the list, right? Haha. So, this idea I have about the medication was damn foolery.*

I have subsequently entertained ideas concerning my fist and his face, which may have resulted in his visiting with a FACE and NOSE specialist. "Nooooo." The stoppage of Ativan had EVERYTHING to do with it.

Finally he says, "I don't think there is anything I can do about this. It could be Meniere's, but it doesn't quite fit." I know that already. It isn't Meniere's; I've already checked that out. Meniere's, the garbage diagnosis when you don't have a clue. Is there a treatment? He says the standard treatment for tinnitus is .5 mg. of Ativan.

What? What did he say? Ativan? Did he actually say that word? The same crap I've been taking? Does he have any freaking idea how upset that makes me? I tell him I don't want any more of that. It doesn't make any sense whatsoever. It's up to me, he says. What is the probability of me taking a medication for all these months and then be

told that a new condition that has suddenly appeared after I
stop taking it is treated with the same GD medication? This
is stupid!

My brain has a hard time accepting this. But what choice do I
have? Still, I DO NOT WANT TO TAKE THAT CRAP AGAIN.
Deep inside me, a powerful intuition tells me not to do it, and tells
me something is terribly amiss here. This intuition or skepticism is
perhaps, in combination with dumb luck and plain old
determination, the thing that will ultimately lead me to the answer
for all that will follow, will help me find the truth, to stumble upon
the website that saved my life: benzo.org.uk and its benzo forum.

> *Then he says the thing that would, at a not-too-distant*
> *point in time, cause me to wonder if I would have to end my*
> *life, a thought so alien to my normal state of mind that I*
> *would never have believed it was possible previously.*
>
> *"You may have to live with this the rest of your life."*
>
> *This GD noise in my head, increasing in both duration and*
> *volume, would be with me the rest of my life? It's already*
> *almost maddening. What if it gets worse? I felt like I had*
> *been punched in the stomach. Hard.*
> *I leave Dr. Demon's, I mean Damon's office in a state*
> *of utter dismay. My stomach does not feel right. Again.*
> *And now I am projecting into a life-long state of screaming*
> *tinnitus.*

It is difficult to explain how frightening those words were. The
thought of living like this for "the rest of my life" sent pure terror
slicing through my being like a knife. The only thing that gave me
relief from that potentiality was the knowledge that I could control
how long "the rest of my life" was to be by simply ending it. Less
than a year ago, I was relatively healthy. Now, I was pondering a
pitiful existence with a not so happy ending.

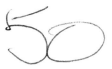

It would get worse, much, much worse. In fact, I would experience, all told, about 50 different symptoms during the next year. That's right, 50, some of which were minor in and of themselves, and some that were beyond brutal all by themselves. The intensity of the tinnitus would become so loud, that at times that I could not hear a person standing right next to me speaking to me. The duration would eventually become constant, 24 hours a day, 7 days a week, save for a few hours of silence about 1 time every month or so. All of the other symptoms would vary in intensity from annoying (if they were by themselves, a single symptom at a time) to horrible, terrible, and ghastly. But there were generally a dozen or more symptoms coexisting. It seems simply unbelievable but it is, as you will see, true.

Simply unbelievable
but it is TRUE.

Live in this world like a stranger, a wayfarer,
and deem yourselves as dwellers of the graves.

-The Prophet Muhammad,
as reported by Ibn Umar

Chapter 13: To Be or Not to Be

Over the next week or two, my anxiety grew like a cancer out of control. It far exceeded the anxiety that I felt during the height of my PTSD, but given that I now had a great deal of past experience at dealing with it, I managed to stay off the drug. It was, however, getting harder and harder not to reach for that bottle filled with .0 mg. tablets of Ativan, remnants of a recent past I wanted to forget. And while the anxiety was blossoming, the tinnitus was, for some reason, suddenly gone. It is all so strange.

I hadn't had any for a while, maybe 2-3 weeks. Maddie was taking a few days to herself, taking her daughter back to the university and hanging around for a few days. I didn't blame her. My moods were deteriorating again, only now nobody knew what was wrong with me. A return of PTSD was ruled out. That made no sense. No intrusive memories. In fact, I had no other symptoms of PTSD at this point except severe anxiety and anger. I also had significant holes in my memory from this time frame, which was actually fine with me.

While Maddie is gone, my anxiety gets even worse, off the GD Richter scale of anxiety. I feel deeply alone. No one knows what is wrong. I keep thinking that no one knows. No one can possibly

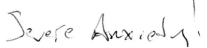
Severe Anxiety!

know. No one understands how powerful this anxiety is. All alone. What has happened to me? I am considering an old friendship. Is she near? I visualize myself turning the steering wheel into the path of an oncoming truck. I give it serious consideration. Suicide.— Serious —

I can't eat. I'm trying. Got to at least have water. Sipping at it, staring at it. Make some soup. Eat 2 or 3 tablespoons. Don't want any more. Feeling of doom, constantly. My stomach is really churning and it won't stop. I can't sit still. Much worse if I do; all I think about is this shitty feeling. Keep walking. Keep moving. Something awful is going to happen, I think. I don't know what. Maybe I'll just go BOOM and explode, pieces everywhere. So what. I look on the internet, type in anxiety. No help. Says to take tranquilizers. That's what I have in that freaking bottle. Shit Prozac *I can't take this. Watch TV. Try distraction. Seinfeld. It's on now. I go find it. I sit and listen. I've seen this one, it's funny. I don't laugh. I can't concentrate on it. This feeling is too powerful. God help me please. Help me Please. Help* distraction *me Please. Tears streaming down my face. Somebody help me. God doesn't want to. Maybe I haven't been good enough. I have tried. That's all I can do, right? Maybe God has nothing to do with this shit. No one to call for help. No one. What can anyone do? Deep breaths. Can't sleep. That's really bad. This is the worst ever. Never this bad before. Why? Why? Why? Something has to give here. Maybe death can be a good friend, after all. I am ready for her to appear. I might have to take one of those goddamn pills. I stare at the bottle. It's still there, on the window ledge by the door. I almost threw it away. No more drugs. No. Not going to take that crap. But I might have to. Nowhere else to turn. GOD HELP ME! I scream it out loud. This is bad, really bad. Tears are streaming down my face. I CAN'T TAKE THIS MUCH LONGER. I walk over to the prescription bottle. Medicine. It IS medicine. Nothing*

to lose, right? It can't hurt? If I take it and it doesn't help,
so what. If it helps, then good.

Finally, after 3 days of unbelievable anxiety and suffering, after
eating almost nothing, I reach down, open the prescription bottle,
and take one of those tiny, 2-mg. tablets of Ativan. Thirty minutes
later, I can take a deep breath with almost no anxiety. Nearly gone.
It helped me. It still helped me. I didn't care about anything else.
Relief. I have never, ever experienced anything like that before. But
at least the medicine still works.

I didn't have a clue then that there was a damn good reason why
it "worked". I was addicted to it. Addicted to a prescription
medication. Me. I was an "addict". Prescription addiction. Only
this "medication", which I should refer to as poison, doesn't let go
so easily. I was soon to have the fight of a lifetime. No, no, not
soon. The fight had already begun, but at this point, I did not know
who the enemy was. *Almost 50*

Prior to the Fall of 2002, having lived for nearly a half-century, I
never really knew what clinical anxiety was. Now, I was living it,
and it is perhaps indescribable. But, for the reader's understanding,
I shall try.

Perhaps we have all experienced waiting for loved ones, a
spouse, older parent, child, partner, and they are very late to arrive
home. A churning begins in the stomach. The clock moves so very
slowly. The churning grows and grows. You can't sit still. You
can't focus on a book or music or the television. You begin to
become consumed with worry. You start pacing, looking out the
window every minute or two. You pray that if the phone rings, it is
not the police telling you about an accident. Your breathing
quickens in pace and shortens in depth. The feeling in your
stomach, high up, is terrible. Where are they? Pacing, breathing
shallow, unable to focus on anything except profound worry, you
stand by the window and look non-stop, hoping that every headlight
will turn into your driveway. You can't take a deep breath. You

can think of nothing else. Your stomach is almost in pain, as worry morphs into something ugly. That feeling in your stomach, one that pervades your entire body, at the very height of your emotions is the closest I can come to describing clinical anxiety. Imagine living like this (but worse) all day, every day, 24/7 "for the rest of your life". Tack on a noise in your head that sometimes blankets all other noise. This was my world. And remember, it gets worse.

it gets worse.

This Medication Doesn't let go so easily (the fight of a lifetime)

Many were empathetic! loud scene!

An old man sits on a granite step.
He plucks a treasured guitar.
The strings throb with feeling;
He needs no audience to open his heart.
A Boy enthusiastically wants to learn his style.
"Style?", asks the old man slowly. "My style is made of
The long road of life, of heartbreak
and joy, and people loved, and loneliness.
Of war and its atrocities.
Of a baby born.
Of burying parents and friends.
My scale is the seven stars of the dipper ,
The hollow of my guitar is the space between heaven and earth.
How can I show you my style?
You have your own young life."

- Deng Ming-Dao

Chapter 14: Searching for Demons

     For the next 2-1/2 months, from September to mid-November, I
would teeter between hope and despair, doggedly determined to
discover the reason for the anxiety and tinnitus. I would take the
Ativan as needed. I would research my symptoms on a regular
basis. Sometimes, tinnitus would appear and rev up over a 2-3
minute period. I would take poison to stop it, and in the beginning it
usually helped. Sometimes, anxiety would spring to life, and I
would take Ativan for it. Most of the time, the poison helped me.
Once in a while, it didn't and I would take a second dose of poison a
few hours later. I also frequently used ice packs on the area near my

ear when the sound gripped me, and thought that maybe it helped a little.

My new job started and I was delighted in spite of the strange cards life had dealt me. Feeding my addiction kept me going. The new environment, free from bullying and conflict, was exciting in many ways. This was a "start-up", a school that, 5 years earlier had begun as a K-2 program and grown by one grade per year. This, my first year at this school but with a long career behind me, was the very first year that there would be a graduating 8th grade class. I was so very excited to be part of this newness. I didn't know how this faculty would measure up to my past school, long recognized as one of the best in the area. In fact, the faculty that the principal, one of the founders of the school, had managed to bring to this new school was outstanding. I was stunned. A perfect blend of new teachers and veterans, all of them filled with boundless positive energy and a willingness to do extra. There were many more leaders in this group than is typical. It is very unusual to find a start-up with this sort of strength in the faculty. And while this school did not have the rich history of success as my previous school, it had experienced a truly meteoric growth. I was very impressed and happy to be there. I felt that I could make a difference here, as the school developed its first ever middle school division.

I was still struggling with in and out anxiety and tinnitus, but was managing these symptoms with the "medication". As time passed, it was helping less and less. Tinnitus was present most of the time, and anxiety was pressing in on me harder and harder. And though I was able to teach, I wasn't completely myself. I faded in and out of clear thinking, but still felt emotionally capable at times.

Within the first week or two of the arrival of students, there arrived another bizarre symptom, one that would stay with me for most of the withdrawal phase of this addiction. I noticed that sound was bothering me. It seemed louder than usual. I couldn't watch TV with anyone at home, at the volume they seemed to prefer. I could not tolerate the radio in the car. At the volume I preferred and thought was appropriate, Maddie couldn't hear it. Odd. This change was happening quickly. The school noise was fast becoming

67

intolerable. I had to close my classroom door all the time. I couldn't understand why students were suddenly being so loud in the classroom. It seemed that lockers were being slammed all the time. Before I realized what was happening, I asked several students why on earth they were slamming their locker. They weren't, of course, but I did not understand. It didn't take long before I realized that the sound meter inside my head was changing and becoming vastly different than it used to be. What seemed normal to everyone else (and previously me, too) now sounded horribly, horribly loud.

Remarkably, something good was also happening, though it was truly an example of a double-edged sword. Not only was my right ear working again, it was working too well. All sound was magnified. Everything seemed louder by a factor of ten. I can tell you that this was extremely uncomfortable; in fact, there was a sort of pain associated with it. It felt like everyone was yelling at the top of their lungs in close proximity to my ears, yet they obviously weren't. I was so happy that my ear was working again, yet it was working in a way that was not pleasant at all.

I had no choice but to go to the Principal and share my woeful tale. She was aware fully of my experience at my previous school, as I had been her daughter's math teacher. She was pleased to have me on board, and she agreed without hesitation to a modification of my responsibilities. Thank God for her. She agreed to remove me from lunchroom responsibilities and I did not have to attend all-school functions. I could not have continued otherwise, and would have again been out of work.

Again, my ENT docs have no understanding of this. They have a name for it: hyperacusis. Labels, they are good at. Causes, they stink at, even though they are specialists. Maybe they are specialists at identifying that people actually HAVE ears, noses and throats, but nothing else. "I'm delighted to tell you that you have the exactly correct ratio of ears to noses to throats. Furthermore, our examination reveals proper location for the aforementioned items." So now I know the names, but I know not the reason for their existence within me. Tinnitus. Hyperacusis. But what on earth is going on? And what on earth is going to happen to me?

I had hyperacusis, anxiety and tinnitus. They were to become my Big Three. Other symptoms would come and go by the dozens. But these three were becoming constant companions. I never knew that hyperacusis existed. Never heard of it before. No one I knew had ever heard of it. Finally, the doctors were openly baffled. No more garbage diagnoses, just shoulder shrugs and honest I don't knows. In the meantime, I was living a nightmare.

In the classroom, I had to make modifications. Sounds were getting louder still. In the past, I had seen an art teacher fashion all of her classroom desk legs with tennis balls, after cutting a small slice in each ball. They fit snugly and they successfully muted sound. That helped. But what about the noise of the students themselves? The hyperacusis was getting so bad so quickly that normal talk was very difficult to deal with and books dropping on desks was nothing short of a bomb attack.

I decided to ask my students for help. One day, abut a week after hyperacusis reared its ugly head, at the start of each of 6 classes, I explained that something had gone wrong with my hearing. When the year started, I had obviously been hard of hearing. Now, that had changed. The ear that used to be "broken" was working again, only it was working too well. I told them that a medication was causing some unpleasant side effects, one of which was "hyperacusis". I wrote the word on the board and explained it. Then I provided a short demonstration. I placed earplugs in both of my ears, positioned so that I could still hear a little. (I had been experimenting with earplugs for several days.) I told them that what sounds normal to them (as I dropped a book onto a desk from about 6 inches up), sounds like this (I slammed the book onto the desk almost as hard as I could) to me. Almost all of the students in each of the 6 classes jumped in their seats at the sound. It worked. They got it. In fact, many of them were empathetic. They took good care of me, especially a group of boys and girls in the 5th grade, who would sometimes glare at the occasional student who forgot and made a loud sound. How lucky I was to have these wonderful students. To this day, I remember their gentle care. Almost every day, someone in one of my classes, fifth through eighth graders, asked me how my ears were. Once in a while, I could manage a humorous response. "Why do you ask? Do they look funny to you?"

Over the next 2 months, well into November, these 3 symptoms would take their toll on me. But I could not stop working. That wouldn't help. As difficult as it was at school, it kept my mind on something other than my plight. I was growing despondent, believing more and more (though not completely) that the demon jerk doctor may have been right, that this was to be my life right to the end. Then, in November, my hyperacusis morphed into something even worse, a pattern that would repeat itself over the next year or so: Terrible things would simply get worse. Suddenly, my own voice sounded 10 times louder. Further, my ears were working like two burnt out speakers whenever I spoke. Buzzing and distorting my own voice, my ears were betraying me. I could not speak with a god-awful distortion buzzing in my head so incredibly loud. This was very, very difficult. I did not want to speak, and did not unless I actually had to. But, of course, I was a teacher. I had no choice. One day, alone in my classroom, behind a closed door, completely depleted, I broke down, tears streaming down my face. I couldn't go on.

Can't talk. Can't sing. No music, no guitar, No humming, no radio, no television. I live alone in my bedroom. No noise. No sound. Can't be with people. They talk. They laugh. I don't. Can't do my job right. Missing things all the time. I can't do this anymore. Pills aren't helping much. Damn noise in my head gets loud, sometimes all day. Goddamn anxiety. Sometimes really bad. And now this. Can't even talk with this giant Goddamn noise in my head, all distorted. Just can't do it. Depleted. Have to quit.

paragraph for 4 pt

can't work

Disappoint Maddie. No more energy. All gone. God. Father, why is this happening to me? Why? Please tell me? Please God. Please, please, please, please, please God help me. Help me, somebody. God, are you there? My stomach. My head. My ears. Can't do this anymore. Got to go tell the boss. Stop crying. Stop it. Just get yourself together.

Deep, deep breaths. Now reconciled to quitting, I slowly pull myself together. My face is dry. I'm ready. As I stand up to walk to the office and resign, I wonder if I can walk that far given what news I was bringing. Maybe I will break down again. What will she say? What *can* she say? I stop briefly before reaching for the doorknob and my mind wanders.

> *I hear the voice of that old friend calling from a distance. I hear my name; a soft whisper from the unknown. I can't make out any other words. I look outside to see where she is. It is only a distant call, but I sense that she is approaching. I know this friend. Perhaps soon she will be with me. I am beginning to think of her more often.*

Just then, perhaps luck, perhaps a Heavenly intervention.

> *A student walks in the room, sits down and quietly prepares for class. Hi, Mr. Mueller. Others follow. I stand there and stare at them. My earplugs are in. They wait patiently for me to move. I take one step, then another. I am not going out the door. Can't leave them here alone. I find myself in the front of the room. The room is completely silent. The students are studying me; they sense something is wrong. I ask with a whisper, "Is everyone's homework out?" My voice buzzes in my head, even with a whisper, but I tolerate it. They nod, all ten of them. They are hard workers. I cannot disappoint them. Thank God I am a veteran teacher. I simply go forward on auto-pilot. No need to plan how to teach something. I can do this with my eyes closed, and do it*

A struggle minute to minute.

well. I just have to talk quietly and hope that the children
will support this odd circumstance. In fact, they do almost
all the time. Thank God. What wonderful kids they are. No
"loud" pranks. They actually care.

On three subsequent occasions over the next few weeks, I break down similarly, completely depleted and overwhelmed by the daily battering world of benzo addiction and withdrawal, fully intending to find my way to the boss's office, and resign. And, miraculously, on each of those three separate occasions someone enters my room or calls on the telephone before I can get out of my room. A student or a colleague, asking for help in some way, stops me every time. Never able to turn down a request for help previously in my life, it is as though people are plotting against me, prohibiting me from completing a task that I feel is inevitable. Conspiracies, real or a product of fantasy, may not always be a bad thing.

Still, I am here, and still, I am suffering. Thankfully, as my mother was 100% Norwegian and I 50%, I am stubborn, or shall I say pig-headed. For even now, deep down inside, I cannot believe, I cannot fully accept that this is to be my existence for the rest of my awful, pitiful life, a life that has become a struggle minute by minute. Time seems to freeze during these times, just when you wish it would move along more swiftly. Funny thing, time is. When you wish it would speed up and the day be done, it sits defiantly still. When life is at its best and you wish to savor every minute, time accelerates. No way is time linear. It plays with us. For now, each day seems like an eternity, with an endless struggle to keep my mind away from how I feel and a constant reminder that my life has fallen apart.

I keep thinking that there must be an answer. There MUST be. I think and think, not quality work, as I am almost constantly under the influence of a tranquilizer, of poison. But I am not going to stop searching. If I do, I surely will die, somehow, with no ship on the horizon, no hope for rescue. Perhaps that old friend will have her way with me regardless. At times, I welcome this notion. But if I keep searching, there is still a molecule of hope.

mother
50%
100%
Norwegian

72

(handwritten: Still on drug & struggling terribly)

(handwritten: God)

> ✣ *We often look to God when we find*
> *our foundations being shaken, only to*
> *find that it is God who is doing the*
> *shaking.*
>
> *-Anonymous*

(handwritten: God)

Chapter 15: Demons Found Alive and Well

November still. My school computer is down. Sitting at my
desk correcting papers, my mind wanders as it does frequently.
Tinnitus, anxiety and hyperacusis are daily demons. I have
stubbornly been cutting the amount of my poison, desperately trying
to wean myself off. My instincts are strong here. I know it is not
good to be on a powerful medication for a long time. But every time
I reach a certain point, symptoms become unbearable. Roaring,
screaming tinnitus, severe hyperacusis, and god-awful anxiety,
which I judge, in the final analysis, to be the worst of all my
symptoms. It's paralyzing, and almost impossible to take your mind
off of. I just have to somehow get off this crap. It HAS to be this
crap. It HAS to be this damn medicine. My logical brain suddenly
re-emerges out of nowhere and kicks into high gear, as it did on rare
occasions, even while drugged. In the past, every attempt at solving
this dilemma failed; thousands of attempts, thousands of failures,
and thousands of deep frustrations. This time, perhaps because of
dumb luck but more likely good old-fashioned determination,
something clicks.

(handwritten: Symptoms become unbearable.)

73

Got to figure this out. I try to take less medicine, my symptoms get worse. What does this mean? What does this mean? What does it mean? Think. Think. ………It still helps, but not as much……… Symptoms always present now. Always. Never a break. How can I keep this up? It almost seems like I MUST take these pills or else. It's almost like……….. an addiction. Addiction? No way. Can't be. Not me! How can it be? I read the goddamn insert. It did not mention the word addiction. <u>Addiction?</u> Is this possible? Gotta find out. Christ. Addiction. Addiction. A wave of fear curses through my body. Addiction? Wait a minute, I think. This is a prescription medication. Yet, I do hear about people being addicted to pain pills. Holy Christ. Maybe it's something similar *to addiction. I don't drink, I don't smoke, I don't do drugs, so how can I have an addiction? Wouldn't be right, would it? Still, it sounds and feels like it might be an addiction. <u>Shit.</u> Maybe it is.*

I stare into space for a few moments, pondering the word "addiction" in half disbelief. The other half of me knows better. My body shivers with anticipation.

I stand up and quickly walk across to my colleague's room. Her computer is working. She is out of the room. She has been a dear friend for many years, having worked through the worst of it at my previous school with me. She left more than a year before me in a similar state to my <u>PTSD.</u> Maybe it was exactly that. She had Andrew's son in her classroom that year. She suffered, too.

Like I have done countless times before, I go to google and type in words for the search. Only this time, I used the words "addiction" and "benzodiazepine". I had never before used this combination of words in a search. Quickly, the search is complete. There, right in front of my eyes, I see one of the "hits":

Benzodiazepine tranquilliser addiction, withdrawal and recovery. Benzo.org.uk

I see it

74

My heart starts to pound. Addiction, withdrawal, and what's that? What's that word? Recovery? What? Recovery? I love the look of that word. Oh my God. Oh my God. I go to the site. This is one of the things that greets me:

> "The biggest drug-addiction problem in the world doesn't involve heroin, cocaine or marijuana. In fact, it doesn't involve an illegal drug at all. The world's biggest drug-addiction problem is posed by a group of drugs, the benzodiazepines, which are widely prescribed by doctors and taken by countless millions of perfectly ordinary people around the world... Drug-addiction experts claim that getting people off the benzodiazepines is more difficult than getting addicts off heroin... For several years now pressure-groups have been fighting to help addicted individuals break free from their pharmacological chains. But the fight has been a forlorn one. As fast as one individual breaks free from one of the benzodiazepines another patient somewhere else becomes addicted. I believe that the main reason for this is that doctors are addicted to prescribing benzodiazepines just as much as patients are hooked on taking them. I don't think that the problem can ever be solved by gentle persuasion or by trying to wean patients off these drugs. I think that the only genuine long-term solution is to be aware of these drugs and to avoid them like the plague. The uses of the benzodiazepines are modest and relatively insignificant. We can do without them. I don't think that the benzodiazepine problem will be solved until patients around the world unite and make it clear that they are not prepared to accept prescriptions for these dangerous products." —Dr Vernon Coleman, Life Without Tranquillisers, 1985.

I am only able to scan, but I feel I may have found the answer. I don't know whether to scream or cry. I am beginning to feel a

Recovery

powerful exhilaration welling up within me. I think I know what is wrong now! I see that there is a forum available. I click and read the welcome. It's all about addiction, withdrawal and recovery. There's that word again, that beautiful, incredible word again. *Recovery*. I hastily figure out how to enroll and make my first "post". I tell whoever is there, somewhere, anywhere the basic story about the Ativan and that I have anxiety and tinnitus. Enter. I'm not sure if I have done it correctly, so I post again within minutes and essentially repeat a brief history. Enter. After 10 minutes or so I see a response. An administrator welcomes me to the site, and tells me that they can help. I am ecstatic. Euphoric. I didn't mention hyperacusis, and I don't know why. Still, I am not convinced completely, not willing to "believe" completely only to feel punched in the stomach if I am wrong. I make a third post focusing on tinnitus and anxiety. I hit enter. Now I am learning a little about how to navigate this place. I see my post. I wait. I hit refresh every 15 seconds. In about 2 minutes, there it is. A response. The most incredible, beautiful, perfect response:

> *Tinnitus and anxiety are 2 calling card symptoms of benzodiazepine addiction and an indication that you are perhaps attempting to withdraw too quickly. Welcome to the forum. We can help you.*

I jump out of my seat. Tinnitus and anxiety are "calling card symptoms"? Really? "We can help you?" Holy crap! I know the answer! They can help me! Holy cow! My eyes well up with tears. I'm smiling and tearful. I know what is wrong! I saw it all there. Recovery. They can help. I sprint back to my classroom and call Maddie, babbling on so fast she cannot understand me. But she hears me say, before I hang up, "I KNOW WHAT'S WRONG!" She can tell I am happy. Actually, I am thrilled beyond comprehension. I know what's wrong. I know what's wrong. I know what's wrong. I know what's wrong. I know what's wrong. I know what's wrong. I know what's wrong. I don't grasp the "more difficult than getting addicts off heroin" portion of the message yet.

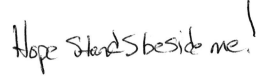
Hope Stands beside me!

It does not matter. I know what is wrong and they can help. I know what is wrong and they can help. Thank you, God. Thank you, God. Thank you, thank you, thank you. My body has goose bumps everywhere. Hope stands beside me for the first time in what seems like an eternity.

Odd, perhaps, that I was exhilarated to discover that I was addicted! That did not matter, initially. I knew what was wrong. For the moment, that is all that mattered.

At some point, I do not remember exactly when, perhaps that day or the next, I swallow hard and ask the BIG question, more specific. I post:

"Will these symptoms ever go away?"

Almost immediately comes the answer, from Jackie. Short, but sweet.

"Yes, Sam. They will."

Praise God. Thank you, Jackie. Tears the size of the Mississippi roll down my face the instant I see those words. "Yes, Sam. They will." Can anyone in the world comprehend how this sounds to my stupid, screwed up ears? I've been living on the edge of madness, pondering a pitiful existence for what seems like an eternity, and now someone is telling me that I will get better. The tears keep coming. I don't know exactly what emotion best fits this feeling. A combination of joy, relief, and renewed hope all there simultaneously, overwhelming me. My cup runneth over. I was lost, but now am found.

In a very short time frame, I went from believing it was a real possibility that my entire future existence forever and ever would be one of constant, unending, suffering to actual, genuine hope that I was going to get better. What a day. What a day.

*Literally thousands of wonderful friends
have accompanied me in life, and many
now await me in the secret eternity to come.
I have enjoyed the long voyage.*

- Ansel Adams

Chapter 16: Benzo.org.uk: Thousands of Members

I am told. · · —

People from all over the world are here. Thousands of members, all at different points in RECOVERY. They are all addicted, and so am I. I am an addict, albeit an accidental addict. Some people here struggle to make their way through the English language. My struggle now is to understand what I have to do. Exhilaration is out the door, and reality is setting in. I am told that this will be the hardest thing I have ever done in my life. I gulp. How can that be? One member posts: "Best of luck to you; this will be the wildest ride of your life!" I'm not sure what that means. I'm not sure about this guy. He isn't encouraging at all. Truth is, I was going to get it straight from these people, whether I liked it or not.

Even though I continue to be more than hopeful, my skeptical side keeps pestering me. Who are these guys, anyway? When I think that, it reminds me of the Lone Ranger. Who was that masked man anyway? That's good, I need a little humor. Yet, the site administrators and moderators are not doctors. A doctor says one thing, they say another. Who is right?

The more I read at the site, the more I was convinced that these people, rather these incredible, beautiful people, who were giving countless hours to helping others, were correct. Within a few days, I experience what feels like a complete lack of doubt. I browse

through what many call "The Ashton Manual", the document for
withdrawal from benzodiazepines, by Dr. Heather Ashton, which
has been made available at the site. The actual name of the
document and the title that Dr. Ashton prefers is *"Benzodiazepines:
How They Work and How to Withdraw".* Her credentials are beyond
outstanding.

Professor C Heather Ashton, DM, FRCP
Emeritus Professor of Psychopharmacology
School of Neurosciences, Division of Psychiatry,
The Royal Victoria Infirmary, Queen Victoria Road,
Newcastle upon Tyne NE1 4LP, England, UK

She has been studying benzodiazepines for over 30 years, and has
been lecturing and writing papers about them for over 20, publishing
over 200 papers. In short, I learn that she is the definitive source on
benzodiazepine withdrawal in the world. The world's foremost
expert! How could I be so lucky? Is this too good to be true?

I begin to read the stories of many forum members. I can't
believe how many of them were similar to mine. Hyperacusis is not
as common as tinnitus and anxiety, but it is there. In fact, anxiety is
found in *every* individual who becomes addicted, and tinnitus was
fairly prevalent, perhaps in 10% of the people whose story I have
read thus far. But what catches my attention soon is the vast number
of different symptoms there are. I can't believe it. The list in the
"Ashton Manual" is unbelievable if not shocking:

Insomnia, nightmares, sleep disturbance
Intrusive memories
Panic attacks
Generalised anxiety, panics and phobias
Sensory hypersensitivity
Depersonalisation, derealisation
Hallucinations, illusions, perceptual distortions

79

Depression, aggression, obsessions
Muscle symptoms
Bodily sensations
Heart and lungs
Problems with balance
Digestive problems
Immune system
Endocrine problems
Fits, convulsions

Now bear in mind that while her list has over 20 symptoms, many of the symptoms that she lists are *general categories*, and that each category can have many sub-symptoms. The complete list? See for yourself (see appendix A, page 168). Only one word comes to mind when I see this list today: staggering. At the time, I do not pay attention to this detail, and I am glad. Otherwise, I may have been more than a little worried. I did not need to know, for example, that *one* of the *many* "bodily sensations" that Ashton includes in her main category is electric shocks. That's right, electric shocks. In this particular category alone there are a couple dozen bizarre and/or just plain terrible symptoms. All I know is that the 3 symptoms I have are God-awful and I have wondered if I were going to go mad and if I should commit suicide. I don't need to know about any more symptoms. I have enough. Soon enough, however, I would find out about those other symptoms. Soon enough.

I also read the story of Ray Nimmo, the founder of this site. I read as much as my confused, numbed brain could read. As a result of his benzodiazepine experience, Ray founded Benzo.org.uk. It has since been recognized as the world's most comprehensive website on benzodiazepine withdrawal. Ray Nimmo's courage and conviction to help others has made him a hero in benzo circles. He's the man, plain and simple. And while he now has let go of his daily responsibility to his benzo forum, which has had a few iterations, he is the spirit behind it all. Ray's site, along with his

Courage & Conviction

fellow administrators and moderators saved my life and has saved countless others.

The forum has experienced several generations of the original one. Ray and most of the original cast of life-savers have moved on with their lives, as they move into varying degrees of healing. Some have healed greatly, others moderately, and still others just enough to reenter that thing called life, that thing that they knew very little of for many years, in some cases. The main website is still there, filled with information, rated the world's most comprehensive site on benzodiazepine addiction and withdrawal. The new and latest forum is called Benzo Island and it continues on with Ray's work.

I should visit Ray's site.
It saved his life.

*Be kind, for everyone you meet
is fighting a hard battle.*

good S -Plato

Chapter 17: The Beginning of the Beginning

So there I was, ready to recover. Just tell me what to do, folks. I remember the main cast of leaders: Ray, James, Jackie, Yvonne, and about 6 more. This was a band of moderators and administrators who would answer questions and give suggestions. They knew more about the practical aspects of withdrawing from benzos than any other group of people in the world. They, too, were scattered around the world, and this made 24-hour coverage of the site possible. Administrators had more power and generally more time at the board. They had the ability to ban unruly members, which happened on occasion. They could answer technical questions about "cutting" (tapering) and provide reassurance. Moderators had similar responsibilities and knowledge and worked with administrators as a team; everyone had different responsibilities. Mods didn't have quite as much technical (computer) responsibility. Yet, all of these people had more extensive knowledge than the members, and knew how to help. Everyone was in the same boat, or had been in the same boat: they were all victims of benzodiazepine addiction. They were all still suffering badly, had moved into a better state of health after their taper was over, or were somewhere in the middle.

I was first instructed to "cross over" to Valium from the benzo I was on. The "crossover" is a series of replacement steps generally over a 4-6 week period to ultimately end up on the equivalent dosage of Valium (diazepam, generically speaking) only. The

Xanax ok worst one

reason for this is that Valium has a very long half-life, which tends to produce a steadier state in withdrawal than other benzos. Further, given the ratio of most of the benzos per mg. to Valium, it is almost impossible to make small enough cuts to the next level. A 10% cut (weekly or every 2 weeks) is considered an aggressive cut, except at very high doses. Try cutting a 2 mg. tablet of Xanax, now the number 1 prescribed benzo, which is equivalent to 40 mg. of Valium *Same cut Kr* by 10% of a pill even once, much less repeatedly. The tablet crumbles. Can't de done. Valium, on the other hand, comes in doses as small as 2 mg., or 1/20 of a Xanax tablet. It is far easier, not hard at all, in fact, to deal with small cuts. For example, to cut from 24 mg. of Valium to 22 mg, all you have to do is take one less 2-mg. pill.

However, I had another issue to deal with. I didn't really know exactly how much Ativan I was on, since I was juggling the dosage as needed and trying to taper down unsuccessfully. I took slightly different amounts every day, a very, very bad thing to do. I now understood why this was so difficult with Ativan. Cutting a 2 mg. tablet dosage by 1/4 of a pill three time a day, for example, means dropping from an equivalent of 60 mg. Valium to 45 mg., a huge 25% cut. It simply does not work. An addicted brain will be angry, something that, in benzo withdrawal, results in very, very unpleasant consequences. The tabs are too small and too concentrated. When I tried to cut down with the Ativan, my body was screaming out for its fix. So I took a day or two to figure this out. Problem solving was time consuming. My cognitive levels were diminished due to the tranquilizing effects of the drug. Essentially, I was trying to determine exactly where my addiction level was. I was lucky, having managed to get myself down to *about* 2-¼ Ativan poison mg. a day. It could have been much worse, all the way up to 6 mg. I had essentially stopped (or rather, TRIED to stop) taking this poison before the addiction level had climbed up that far.

I decided to use that as a basis. 2.25 mg. of Ativan poison = 22.5 mg. of Valium. Since I wasn't exactly sure, I added a wee bit and decided to "cross" to 24 mg. of Valium, an extra security measure. A cross to Valium and then a slow taper is by far the best vehicle for

22.5 √

what is phenobarbital,

recovery from addiction. It turned out to be exactly where I belonged, a combination of some careful, drugged thought and luck.

There was, however, still *another* major hurdle ahead, one that many victims *cannot* successfully clear. I had to convince my GP that this was the way to go. I had kept him apprised of everything. He is an unusual doctor, actually possessing substantial knowledge of Eastern Medicine and alternative approaches to illnesses in general. I called his office and left a message. He returned the call quickly, as I had labeled my message as urgent. I hurriedly explained my discoveries. He listened. My articulation was weak and somewhat chaotic. I did a poor job. He was skeptical, since it was and still is common medical practice, once a benzo addiction is identified, to either:

1. go the inpatient approach, completely and suddenly remove the patient from benzos, substitute a non-benzo and/or add Phenobarbital as a guard against seizure and death, or

2. taper off the current benzo directly as an outpatient in about 3 – 6 weeks, which is very unwise, too. Depending on the dosage prior to this fast taper, seizures are also possible. It is almost impossible to taper directly off of one of the more powerful benzos such as Xanax and Klonopin (1 mg. of these benzos is equivalent to 20mg. of Valium).

Ass backest

One critical point must be made about these two approaches. Both are more likely to result in long-term symptoms that can go on far past the final dose and perhaps indefinitely. Both approaches yield far more suffering. I have spoken with several benzo sufferers who were treated via the inpatient approach. Their stories are beyond hellish, and their symptoms exist for years and possibly forever. (This is called protracted withdrawal.) The mere mention of that phrase to anyone at the website revs up fears exponentially. It is akin to being a character in a Harry Potter book and saying "Voldemort". No, it's much worse, because life is non-fiction the last time I looked.

Protracted withdrawal

84

Anyway, I am clear-thinking enough to understand/sense that my Doctor is not jumping on board. I simply cannot find the right words. I have to think fast. I ask him if he will accept a fax, which will explain the rationale much better. I send him the following portion of the Ashton Manual:

THE WITHDRAWAL

(1) Dosage tapering. There is absolutely no doubt that anyone withdrawing from long-term benzodiazepines must reduce the dosage slowly. Abrupt or over-rapid withdrawal, especially from high dosage, can give rise to severe symptoms (convulsions, psychotic reactions, acute anxiety states) and may increase the risk of protracted withdrawal symptoms (see Chapter III). Slow withdrawal means tapering dosage gradually, usually over a period of some months. The aim is to obtain a smooth, steady and slow decline in blood and tissue concentrations of benzodiazepines so that the natural systems in the brain can recover their normal state. As explained in Chapter I, long-term benzodiazepines take over many of the functions of the body's natural tranquilliser system, mediated by the neurotransmitter GABA. As a result, GABA receptors in the brain reduce in numbers and GABA function decreases. Sudden withdrawal from benzodiazepines leaves the brain in a state of GABA-underactivity, resulting in hyperexcitability of the nervous system. This hyperexcitability is the root cause of most of the withdrawal symptoms discussed in the next chapter. However, a sufficiently slow, and smooth, departure of benzodiazepines from the body permits the natural systems to regain control of the functions which have been damped down by their

[Handwritten top margin: reinstatement of brain function takes a long time!]

presence. There is scientific evidence that reinstatement of brain function takes a long time. Recovery after long-term benzodiazepine use is not unlike the gradual recuperation of the body after a major surgical operation. Healing, of body or mind, is a slow process.

The precise rate of withdrawal is an individual matter. It depends on many factors including the dose and type of benzodiazepine used, duration of use, personality, lifestyle, previous experience, specific vulnerabilities, and the (perhaps genetically determined) speed of your recovery systems. Usually the best judge is you, yourself; you must be in control and must proceed at the pace that is comfortable for you. You may need to resist attempts from outsiders (clinics, doctors) to persuade you into a rapid withdrawal. The classic six weeks withdrawal period adopted by many clinics and doctors is much too fast for many long-term users. Actually, the rate of withdrawal, as long as it is slow enough, is not critical. Whether it takes 6 months, 12 months or 18 months is of little significance if you have taken benzodiazepines for a matter of years.

[Handwritten left margin: comfortable for me. ✗]

[Handwritten left margin: rate of withdrawal is not critical as long as it is slow enough.]

I send it immediately. I wait. He is very busy, I know that. Highly regarded, he is the senior physician at this practice. An eternity, for certain, passes. About 2 hours later, he calls.

> *"Okay, Sam. It makes sense. I'm willing to give this a shot. Are you ready for the long haul? This isn't going to be fast. Are you certain you are ready for this?"*

I think I say thank you several million times,
perhaps even a gazillion times. To keep
matters simple, I ask for the generic version
of Valium, diazepam, 8-mg. t.i.d., using 2 mg.
tablets only. That means I will be taking 12
tablets a day, once we achieve the cross, but
the ease of cutting that I will have was most
critical.   why havent I totally crossed?

   Some people can tolerate a faster cross than others.
While these are all classified as benzodiazepines, each of
them has a slightly different profile. Ativan is intended more
for anxiety, while Valium is more for sleep. I am told to
expect a higher level of sedation during and after the cross,
for about 3 weeks or so. As always, they are right. Six
weeks is the recommended time frame for crossing to
Valium. I am able to cross, step by step, every 3-5 days or
so, in about 3 weeks. This is faster than many people can
tolerate, but three weeks is doable by some people. This
desire of mine to push forward was going to be a big
problem. The first step of the cross has me worried as I feel a
little disoriented, but then it is "fine". All the while, my
symptoms persist. But for now, spurred on by the thrill of
my discovery of a potential path to good health again, they
seem to bother me less psychologically.

   My cross begins on November 16, 2003, and takes me to Friday,
December 5. I am now taking four 2-mg. tablets of Valium 3 times
a day. This will absolutely knock out most people, but I am
addicted, and have built up a resistance to the effects of the drugs.
The highest daily Valium equivalent dosage of Ativan and Klonopin
I was on was 100 mg., or 50 of these little bastards. Even now I
think, "Holy Crap" at that thought. After I finish the cross, I have to
stay at this level for a week, giving my body plenty of time to adjust
to the new benzo. I feel pretty good during this week. My symptom
level drops to a more manageable level, especially the anxiety and

tinnitus. Manageable………..what a word. Let the reader not misunderstand. It does not mean I feel good. I still feel horrible, but it is a lesser horrible, a level that did not make me feel like dying. That I feel "better" during this week is perhaps due to two reasons. First, Valium generally produces a steadier state because of its longer half-life. Or, perhaps, I have crossed to a Valium dosage that is just above my actual addiction level. My addiction is being fed properly, steadily. Looking back, I think both were true. No matter, I feel better, and I am ready to cut, ready to roll, and *ready to get done with it*. Even though I have read *not* to rush, it has not yet sunk in. Seems to me this will be simple. I devise a schedule of weekly cuts, quite aggressive, that will get me off of this poison in about 3 months. I can't wait to feel GOOD again. I haven't felt well in a long time. Just like severe, chronic pain, there is only so much we can take before we decide to take catastrophic action.

While the good turn of events (the discovery of my addiction and course of action towards recovery) has pushed memory of my old friend to the deep recesses of my mind, she still lurks there, waiting to be called. She means either suicide or—

The basic principle during the slow taper is to make cuts small enough so that your body gets "fooled", and doesn't fully recognize that you are slowly but surely cheating it out of its fix (steady tissue concentrations). Given Valium's long half-life, this makes perfect sense to me, and I am fully ready to fool myself. I'm not going to even think that I have made a cut. I think I am being pretty clever.

The general guideline for cutting is a 10% cut or lower (10% is bold and generally too aggressive in practice) every 1 to 2 weeks, preferably lower except at very high doses. Additionally, the Ashton Manual called for cuts every 1-2 weeks. At the forum, however, 1-week cuts were not common. For the most part, the forum was populated with people who had already tried to stop and couldn't (like me), or really long term users. One of my friends there took Ativan for over 30 years. She disappeared from the forum as she approached lower doses, a time frame which can, in some cases, be brutal magnified by infinity. I planned to push the envelope as

88

He's pushing the envelope.

much as I could. I think I can hear God laughing as I write that, or maybe it's just me laughing at my previous self.

> *And so it begins. On December 12, 2003, I make my first cut from 24 mg. of Valium to 22mg. I am so, so excited. I'm on my way. Hallelujah. Thank you, God. I am so fortunate to have found benzo.org.uk. I have been taking 8 mg. of Valium, t.i.d. (four 2-mg. tablets each time) for 1 full week after my cross, a total of 24 mg. of Valium daily. I feel very sedated, which is probably a good thing. I cut 2 mg. from my midday dose, as recommended. I am a tiny bit nervous, but determined. While I am enthused, I can't see the road ahead. Thank God. Thank God.*

- addiction.

"This isn't a Race."

- James

Chapter 18: Who are you Kidding?

December 12. The midday dose is now 3 tabs. I am off to a good start. No problems. They said at the site that some people "feel" a cut within hours. I wonder what that means. The next 2 days are uneventful, still with steady, moderate tinnitus, moderate anxiety and stupid loud hyperacusis. Moderate is not to be misunderstood. If the reader were suddenly to experience this, it would feel extreme, unbearable and cause enormous fear. But I was used to it to some degree. I had to be; I had no other reasonable, rational choice.

This isn't bad at all. Jeez, I didn't "*feel*" anything at all. Maybe this wasn't going to be that bad after all…… "moderate" symptoms I can deal with most of the time.

December 15 arrives. Maddie is shaking gently shaking me, trying to wake me with her typical softness. I give a little smile. I feel okay. Then, within seconds, the act of awakening overloads my hyper-stimulated nervous system.

> *Holy shit, Oh My God……It's LOUD…screaming in my head sounds like a jet engine. God tell me this isn't so. Please no no no no no no no no no. BLOCK IT OUT! DON'T THINK ABOUT IT! Need help……gotta make a post. I start to get up. And what's this? What's this? My*

90

Like a
band
w/o effect.

*head feels like it is in a vise. Something is squeezing it and it feels like warm metal. Holy crap, this is intolerable. Pressure all around my head. Never felt this before. Am I having a stroke? Maybe. No, no, no. I can move and talk. Both hands feel strong. Oh my God the sound is horrendous. Worse than horrible. What am I gonna do? Somebody help me. Turn off that noise! What is going on? What the F? I want to smash my head open. Smash it! Crush it! Is this how it is going to be? This is beyond horrible. I have to smash my head open. God Almighty. Can't do this, can't do it, **can't do it**! But I have to do it. **I have to**! Concentrate. Get online. Ask. Concentrate. I'm really scared. Scared as hell. Get online. Get online.*

Maddie asks if she can help, and I yell NO as loud as I can without blowing out my burn-out speaker ears and head wide open, brains on the wall. She walks away frightened.

I quickly get online and make a post. Help, I ask. 4th day of a cut, I woke up and I feel really bad. Tinnitus loud, loud, head pressure bad. A metal band is pressing on my head. Pain is awful, terrible. All around. Is this normal? Help. The response comes in about 5 minutes.

Yes, this is called "feeling" a cut. Not unusual at all. Especially in the morning, things can get very bad, Sam, as you are revving up your body systems. Generally, this type of response passes slowly as the day goes forward or maybe by the next day or two. Hang in there. This is normal.

this is normal

Normal? Bullshit. What? What do they mean, normal? Normal for what? Normal for who? Oh, Christ, now I know what that guy meant by "quite a ride". Jesus, he was right. I write back…

Me: Maybe this is a stroke or something. Like a brain tumor.

Forum: No, Sam, not a stroke. Not a tumor. This very common. Hang in there. Focus on something. Distract yourself. It can't hurt you. It will pass.

Can't hurt me? How can this not hurt me? When will it pass? I can't take this very long. Distract myself? Jesus, I thought I was going to fool my brain, trick it. Some goddamn trick. THAT'S out the freaking window.

I had, in fact, read something about trying to find as many distractions as possible, things that I like to do, hobbies.

What an I do? Can't do guitar, as the sound would likely kill me dead. Can't sing. Nothing with sound. Cards. The only thing I can do that is nearly soundless is cards. I can play cards. But how the hell can that help? I don't know what to do. Have to get to school. Friday. Shower. Maybe shower will help. God something has to help, something!

Shower does not help. Water on my head sounds like little bomblets. Have to push through it. Got to brush my teeth.

I am scared, really scared. This is bad, really bad. I can't go on like this. The sound in my head, everything in the world is so horribly loud, anxiety is unbelievable, much worse than ever, a million times worse than it ever was. Now this damn pressure and heat on my head. Christ I can hardly move my head. The pain is bad, really bad.

I am desperate. I go to the freezer and grab a flexible icepack. I'm ready to go, just want quiet. Leave me alone. I sit in my trusty chair and press the ice pack against my right ear/jaw area hoping to numb this shit somehow. About 15 minutes later, there is some relief, not much, but some. I take the icepack with me and I'm off to school. How will I do my job today? Don't know. I'll just do it,

92

somehow. My eyes fill with tears. I feel like I am in a nightmare, a living nightmare.

  Simultaneously, I wonder how on earth I am ever going to do this taper thing, maintain a teaching job, keep my marriage together, not lose my house, etc. while at the same time ponder the fact that the icepack did actually make a small difference. I have to solve that little puzzle, as it may hold an answer of some sort. Can't do it now, though.

> *Maddie can't take much more. If I really love her and want to keep her in my life, I simply have to push forward. I've got to believe in these people at benzo.org.uk, a complete pack of strangers. Most of them live across the pond, with a few based in the U.S. and Australia. What if they are all a bunch of psychos brought together by a common psychosis? Oh, man I'm buying into a den of lunatics! No. no. no. I've read the website carefully. These are real, bright, articulate people who have been in my shoes, and in some cases still are. They can help, I know it. What are my choices, really? Stop being so fearful, Sam. Push forward. Push forward. You must.*

I hear her now, pretty clearly. She is getting closer. She is calling me; she just wants to talk. Or am I subconsciously calling her? "Go to hell where you belong", I tell her. There is a pained look on her face. I've hurt her. I feel bad. But I don't want her here. Get the hell away. You'll have your day in the sun. Someday. Not now. Not yet. She is a friend to all of us, I think.

  Over the next 5 months or so, I played solitaire thousands of times. It did distract me. I was taught to play card games as a young boy. Hearts, Pinochle, Bridge. I was playing bridge, though not so well, at age 11. I liked these games. They were challenging, particularly Bridge, in a class by itself. I played hearts against the computer a million times. I played chess against the computer, but I could not gather my game to compete against even the novice level.

93

I played poker with pretend opponents. Every possible card game that I remembered (dozens) I played, sometimes with Maddie. My cognitive abilities were significantly impaired and I knew it.

I did everything I could to remove my focus and energy from myself and the gathering and growing storm. Soon, I would have so many symptoms that I would lose track of how many. I stopped counting. It didn't matter. The only thing that mattered was staying resolute in getting off this poison.

I could easily have been assessed as being mentally ill by someone who had no knowledge of my symptoms and only my behavior. I wanted to be alone. No sound. No questions. No talking. Just get online and be where they understood me. They understood my invisible demon of a friend; she was after them, too.

invisible demon of a friend.
Death by
suicide.

We have nothing to fear but fear itself.

- Franklin D. Roosevelt

Chapter 19:   Fear

Fear was a fearless "friend" for much of this journey, a
companion to my friend of final peace. During my time with PTSD,
while I did have aggressive times as described in earlier chapters,
when I was not aggressive, I was fearful. In fact, the aggressiveness
that I displayed was my way of dealing with my underlying fears.
Either I would cave in to them and be fearful, or I would defy them
and become an aggressive type. Fight or flight, it seems, is a real,
existing dichotomy, not just psychobabble.

During the vast majority of my PTSD experience, I was fearful. I
was afraid of accidentally running into one of the principles in the
drama, perhaps afraid of letting go with a few, quick left jabs and
then a right cross, or afraid that I might just turn away and start
running. Either was possible. To this day, I am uncomfortable
entering the town where my first school resides. I was embarrassed
that I could not remember about 50% of the names in my life and
large segments of time: my students, colleagues, past students,
events, etc. I would, upon occasion, find myself face-to-face with
one or two of them in the grocery store after hearing, "Hi, Sam!", or
"Hi, Mr. Mueller!", and, unable to recognize who they were, would
simply stare at them trying in vain to remember the voice, the face,
the posture, something, anything. How awful. I would simply say,

Memory loss.

"I'm sorry, I'm having trouble with my memory right now." It was terribly embarrassing, but I was doing the best I could.

During conversations with former colleagues, I was inevitably and politely reminded that I had already mentioned one thing or another to them. I was shocked, since I had absolutely no recollection of seeing them or speaking with them. Occasionally, I would find humor in this circumstance, looking at a friend that I knew quite well, being told that she had stopped over at my house and had extended conversation with me, but I simply could not remember it. There is something funny about that, and I would laugh about it sometimes. Mostly, I was embarrassed.

There were triggers, that is to say, words or names or places that would cause me to be suddenly irate, a response to an underlying fear. But for the most part, there was just plain old fear. This fear was a direct result of and part of the psychiatric brain injury known as PTSD.

Please, please, please, if you ever hear someone referring to a soldier's PTSD as an "emotional problem", particularly someone in the armed forces, perhaps an official spokesman, who is allegedly trying to be helpful, promise that you will stand up and tell this person that if they ever use that phrase again relative to a soldier's PTSD that you will sock them in the head. Get their attention. Then explain slowly and carefully that referring to a soldier's PTSD as an "emotional problem" is demeaning and diminishing. It mocks them. Never let this happen. It is a classified injury to the brain. The soldier has NO control over it. You can't just knuckle down, buckle down, suck it up, shoulders back, stomach in and get over it, any more than you could magically make a broken arm better. It is an *injury*.

Since my experience with complex PTSD, a variety of classic PTSD that is shorter in duration, I have seen many news stories about our men and women returning from the Iraq War, our president's senseless, theocon vehicle of mass-murder, having difficulties such as PTSD. The military generally mistreats these soldiers, despite what they say. It is perceived as a weakness, an emotional inability to deal with war. That is categorically not the

case. This version of PTSD is tough to deal with. There is no
guarantee that healing will take place in a year or two. Suffering can
last much longer. To suggest that these men and women are having
emotional difficulties is ignorance at its worst. These men and
women set out to do what they perceived as a good thing, their
patriotic duty. I would argue that this was, in this case, this war,
misguided thinking, but that matters not. Suggesting that their PTSD
is a weakness/emotional problem is a seriously mean-spirited shot in
the back.

But back to fears. Fear is one of the predominate aspects of
benzodiazepine addiction and withdrawal. It is not an aspect of
one's personality. It is, quite simply, drug (poison) induced. Every
single person in true benzo withdrawal can find themselves at the
mercy of drug-induced fear, and they fight a ferocious battle to stave
off defeat. For defeat will only mean a constant, endless self-
examination of symptoms, every waking moment, always feeling
certain that each new symptom heralds the onset of a terminal
illness. It would mean the creation of the mother of all
hypochondriacs. And, above all, it would cause, without doubt, a
significant ratcheting-up of symptoms, an endless cycle of physical
and psychological battering of self.

Fear is ever-present in withdrawal, and every day the person in
withdrawal must beat it off with a stick, lest they become sicker.
And while it is almost impossible to completely win this battle, it is
possible to win most small victories every day, eventually winning
the war.

One of the positive lessons the benzo sufferer learns, in the end,
is that we are capable of withstanding far more than we ever
imagined we could. Our well is far deeper than we realized, and we
are stronger than we ever believed.

To give you some idea of the extent that fear enters the life of
someone in benzo addiction and withdrawal, here is a list of some
actual things, very simple things that I was fearful of, not just a little
afraid, but nearly terrified of at times:

it is possible to win
most small victories every
day, eventually winning
the war.

- the telephone
- someone knocking on the door
- being asked to place or do the dishes
- the upcoming holidays
- ✓ leaving my bedroom
- strangers
- some foods (crunchy)
- crowded rooms
- the future
- ✓ doing something new
- the radio *why*
- the television *why*
- going into a store
- going out to dinner
- getting a hair cut
- ✓ leaving my bedroom (repeated intentionally)
- being asked to do anything

need intense @ home.

Most of my free time was spent in my private bedroom and solitary world, and at benzo.org.uk. It was the only place I found comfort, and even here, there were times of enduring difficulty. When we are suffering, we often find comfort only with those who truly understand, and while in benzo withdrawal, only those taking the same journey, those like you, who became accidentally addicted to the hellish poison called benzodiazepines can be considered fellow travelers. The entire list of symptoms is invisible. No one can see what's wrong with you, but it is real, a true living nightmare.

If you live in constant fear of something, even be it the unknown, it pervades your entire existence. In fact, the unknown may be the worst of all! It magnifies everything by many factors of ten. I remember vividly a member of the forum writing a post about the agonizingly deep horror he felt when he accidentally killed a very small moth in his home. He was trying to catch it and put it outside (as I would do), but as moths can be very delicate, it was

no one can see what's wrong with you.

98

accidentally killed. He was devastated and could not post at all for a few days. To him, it was as though the world has experienced a cataclysmic event. Sadness had been magnified exponentially. And so it is in withdrawal from benzos. The television news cannot be tolerated. Any bad news is shunned. Otherwise, our lives feel unlivable. And not far down the road, in January, I was to experience my own cataclysmic event, a sadness so profound that I cannot think of it even today without fighting back a flood of tears. At the time, I thought the world would surely end, and I profoundly wanted it to. It was the worst day of my life, and soon thereafter that old friendship grew close again, closer than ever.

Any bad news shunned!.

Do not make a schedule to for into the future. [handwritten]

Never try to teach a Pig to sing. It wastes your time and just annoys the pig.

you do i.d... [handwritten]

-anonymous

Chapter 20: Happy Holidays (December)

After that first cut, I had to quickly reevaluate my expected course. I had been warned not to make a schedule too far into the future, especially in the beginning. But I chose to ignore that warning, believing that I was somehow different or stronger. I was neither.

Day 4 of my first cut was the worst day I had symptomatically since that late October morning over a year earlier when everything began falling apart. December 15, a Monday, is an opportunity to be humble, to learn. My symptoms do diminish a small amount during that day, but remain essentially horribly high. I remember wondering if I felt a tiny bit better or if I was only getting used to these hideous symptoms. I force my way through the day by spending every free minute in between classes at the forum. I ask many questions, and get answers I don't like.

the forum - Benzo.org uk [handwritten]

Sam: Am I going to feel like this throughout the taper?
James: No, Sam, every day will be different. Your symptoms will come and go, rise and fall. There is an ebb and flow to withdrawal, but one thing you can count on: there is no pattern. One symptom will fade while a new one appears.

There is no pattern : this A bumpy ride [handwritten]

100

I don't fully accept or understand the new symptom part. And I try to make predictions about which day will be worse. Why? I want to be prepared. However, I have been told that's not how it works. The only predictable element of benzo withdrawal is the tremendous unpredictability. I am hoping that weekends will be *he's working* worse than weekdays, so I don't have to push my way through a work day. Not wishing to have the experience of the 15th repeated, I alter the pace of my taper, and decide to make the next cut in 2 weeks, on December 26, after the Christmas festivities. I am very fearful of the holiday gatherings, as I know they will place me in the middle of wanting to act well for Maddie and having to deal with ungodly sound levels, being forced to talk above the pitch of the crowd, causing miserable buzzing in my head from my own voice, etc, etc, etc. And all those fears lead to heightened anxiety.

The vise-like grip around my head subsides somewhat. Tinnitus drops a little, too, for a few days. Anxiety is always there, wearing away at my energy, a daily assault. Then on day 9 and 10 of this cut, I am certain I have the flu. When I wake up in the morning, it is 90 minutes or so before the alarm. I feel flushed, warm, and ache all over. My stomach feels like I have to run a mile. I ask about this, believing I have the flu. No, Sam, this is a common side effect. It will pass.

The flue - common side effect

Jesus! They keep saying everything will pass. Is that all there is to say? Will I keep getting new symptoms? The answer is: most likely. Crap!!! When will the old ones go away? No one knows. There are no patterns to be found. James tells me this more than once. But things will ultimately get better. They keep telling me this. I must believe it or I will turn the wheel in front of an oncoming truck.

Things ultimately will get better!

The metal band around my head begins to blend into this flu-like state. Tinnitus flares up and down throughout these 2 days from hour to hour. I am helpless. Except for an occasional ice pack, which still seems to help a small amount, it just has a life of its own. I can't figure that out. Hyperacusis is still here. I continue waking up about 90 minutes before the alarm sounds with adrenaline surges in my stomach, a very odd, uncomfortable feeling that makes me want to run ten miles.

Mealtime is very difficult. I cannot eat in the lunchroom at school. At home, Maddie is walking on eggshells. If she accidentally touches 2 ceramic plates together while cleaning up after dinner, I glare at her like she has committed a major criminal offense, a felony. The penalty for this crime is death by staring. God forbid that she asks ME to do this task. I am NOT volunteering, no way. When she gets tired of doing everything herself, she asks for my help. *I don't want to do it!* Those freaking dishes will kill my head for sure.

> *Forum: Hyperacusis is very unpleasant, Sam, but it cannot actually hurt you.*

When I do the dishes, I move in slow motion, almost like a mime. It takes me forever. I cannot let the silverware fall from my hand even an inch away from their final resting place. Everything must be carefully *placed* down. The truth is that this is exactly the sort of task I need, and Maddie knows it. It forces me to use extreme concentration and causes me to be distracted from my bizarre little universe.

Over time, I have noticed something odd about my tinnitus. Whenever I bend over toward the floor, my tinnitus increases drastically as though someone has their finger on a volume knob. I ask about this at the forum. No one has heard about anything like this. For others at the site, tinnitus is a constant, changing only from day to day slightly or from week to week, or unbelievably, never changing at all. Most people at the forum who have tinnitus have bilateral tinnitus. Mine is only in my right ear. This positional tendency of mine is growing worse it seems. I cannot lie flat in bed. When I do, the volume goes up several notches. I can't drown out the sound with music like others can, since I have hyperacusis. A rather unfortunate combination. I get an old, worn reclining chair from the basement and carry it up the stairs by myself. In the bedroom it goes, and this will be my new bed for about 6 months. It allows me to "recline" while still keeping my head up somewhat. I quickly adjust to this chair and sleep through the night, save the occasional potty trip, until my adrenaline surges wake me.

Thank God for this sleeper tendency of mine. I can fall asleep through medium tinnitus. When it gets really bad, I use an icepack and often fall asleep with the side of my head against it.

The sound quality of my tinnitus is emerging as multi-tonal. There are several distinct sounds. One is a jet engine. Another is a combination of loud bacon frying together with popcorn popping. The third sound I hear is a generator, lower in pitch than the jet engine. There are more, but I cannot describe them. More than a positional quality, there also seems to be a relationship to my old TMJ (temporo-mandibular joint syndrome) issue, which hasn't surfaced since my mid-twenties. I discover that different jaw positions cause a change in the quality and volume of my Tinnitus. When I push in on my jaw or open really wide, there is a *distinct* change in pitch and volume. No one else at the forum experiences this. Everyone else with tinnitus finds no change in it's pitch; it is steady, 24/7. Some tinnitus sufferers find that the volume changes with the time of day. Waking often produces an increase in the volume, as the body systems become more stimulated. Others, mostly those who have had tinnitus for longer periods, years after they tapered off benzos, find that nothing changes ever, day after day, 24/7. It is possible that they are in protracted withdrawal and may never experience much improvement.

My doctor suggests that acupuncture can help with the anxiety and even tinnitus, though the tinnitus relief will be more temporary. I am willing to try anything, and although I have read fascinating stories about acupuncture, I am a little skeptical.

I have heard of Carol before. The mother of a former student of mine, she has a tremendous reputation as an holistic healer through nutrition (a macrobiotic approach), acupuncture and essential oils. I have no idea what the hell essential oils are, and I really don't care.

I just want some relief, please, please, please. Nothing else was working, and I was, well, "skeptically open-minded".

My first appointment with her is on a Tuesday afternoon, right after school is over, at 4:00. It is a 40-minute drive that takes me only minutes from my home. It is also day 12 of my first cut. I am not doing so well, but not as badly as day 4. Day 9 and 10 also find me with a "response" to the first cut, but again, not as severe as day 4. On my first visit, she takes a long medical history. She examines my tongue. She smells my stomach. She takes my pulse and explains that there are different types of pulses. She presses my arms in a few places, such as at my elbow, on the inside, thumb side with my arm in the anatomical position. Ouch. Tender. Then she presses on my wrist, about 2 inches below my thumb. Same thing; it is very sore. This surprises me. She nods her head. "Strong anxiety". Finally, I lie down on her table. My socks come off and I am ready. My feet are clean, I think. Geez, I hope so; I haven't been paying much attention to my feet. They seem so distant! Carol tells me that before the acupuncture session begins, she would like to see how responsive I am to some oils that she will prepare, oils that are intended to help me relax. I watch her as she places 2 different oils in the palm of one hand and mixes them. She rubs some on my upper chest and dabs a little around my nose. Very nice smell, I learn it is a combination of juniper and helichrysom. She asks me how I feel about the smell; is it pleasant or unpleasant? I tell her it is very pleasant. But, inside, I wonder how this is going to help, and some pangs of regret enter into my thinking. How on earth can smelly oils do any good? It seems so silly that I almost chuckle out loud.

> *Is she a witch doctor or something? How are smelly oils going to help me for God's sake? I thought this was an acupuncture session not smell class. Smell class, that's funny. Hahahahahaha.*

She asks me to take some slow deep breaths through my nose to take in this pleasant if not silly fragrance. Then she tells me she is going to touch my right ear, the really screwed up one with the tinnitus. What happens next is so surprising and unexpected to me that I almost come out of my skin in shock. The instant, and I mean the *instant* that she touches the rim of my ear with this oil mixture something miraculous happens. My tinnitus changes pitch (lower) and drops off the table to a very low level, still audible, but lower than it has been in centuries (seems that way). It is as though she found the volume switch. I was not expecting this. I have to work hard not to sit up and shout Halleluiah. I find myself saying, "What the hell!? What did you do?"

> *What the hell was that? How can touching my ear possibly do that? I don't understand the connection. What's the physiology? What's the mechanism? It doesn't make any sense. But frankly, I don't give a damn how it worked! HA! It just did, and I don't care how.*

Carol asks me to describe what I felt. I tell her, and she smiles. I'm smiling broadly. We're both happy. Relief, even if it is to be temporary. Relief. Thank you God and thank you Carol.

The acupuncture drops my anxiety level down several notches as well. I am feeling some blessed relief for the first time in a long time, though still with an array of other symptoms. While delighted, Carol does not know how long the relief will last. It doesn't matter. I have some relief. This is as close to joy as I can experience right now.

I subsequently learn in an article about acupuncture that in some pilot studies, acupuncture for prisoners addicted to drugs such as crack, heroin, etc. has been far more effective than traditional approaches. And I learn that one of the key areas is the rim of the ear!

When I arrive home I am smiling for the first time in a long, long time. Maddie gives me a big hug and I tell her the whole story, slowly and with great dramatic flare, right through the cursed hyperacusis, which remains unchanged. I am feeling a little better for now.

I am still feeling better on Wednesday, Christmas Eve day, though the Tinnitus and anxiety are slowly returning to previous levels. I decide not to wait until Friday to make the next cut. I am impatient, even after my first cutting experience. At noon, I take only 2 Valium tablets, thus reducing my total dosage to 20 mg. My dosing is now 8-4-8, morning, noon and evening. In terms of a percentage, this is *only* a 9% cut. However, my first cut was about 8%. It is slightly higher in terms of percent. Since I am feeling a little better as a result of the acupuncture, I have some confidence that I will not respond to this cut the same way as the first. But that extra one percent also has me thinking.

A good portion of this experience, I suppose, depends on individual personality differences as they relate to the ability to tolerate this "ride". Two people with exactly the same symptoms can have a very different response to them emotionally and how they express the experience.

My self-talk and my public expression at benzo.org.uk were worlds apart. My self-talk was far more real than my controlled, public persona. I felt a significant amount of guilt, since my symptoms, though horrible enough, seemed less severe than some of those being articulated at the forum. There were people who had unending body vibrations 24/7, screaming bilateral tinnitus 24/7, electrical shocks cursing through their bodies frequently throughout the day, people with indigestion and acid reflux so bad that they were doubled over a good portion of the time, people with severe muscular pain so bad that they could not walk, many people bed-bound, and on and on. Sometimes, people who were violently suffering simply vanished from the website. Sometimes they returned. A few times they did not. As I ultimately became a moderator, I learned that there were some instances when benzo sufferers simply could not go on in spite of the support and advice at the board. They disappeared intentionally, falling victim to their own hands: suicide. This information, understandably, was not shared with the general board. Given all this, how could I, gifted with the ability to somehow continue working, possibly find a way to complain? I chose to overstate the positive and not report many of my symptoms as well as their severity.

There was another reason for this. I very deliberately stored every possible symptom that was discussed on the board in my memory banks. I worked hard at this. The reason, to me, was quite simple and logical. With this simple effort, I would not be overly consumed by the fear aspects of new symptoms if I knew them to be "normal" for this experience. It worked beautifully. Almost every new symptom that piled on, I had heard of. It didn't change the symptoms, but it did alter my fear response to them. And I came to learn that this was critical, as fear itself was known to ratchet up symptoms *all by itself*!

After trying to surprise myself again with an unexpected cut on the 24th, I wondered what would happen, but kept my mind off of this concern as much as possible. I limped through Christmas without incident, except the typical disappearing act I pulled on multiple instances when company was present in the house. The more time I could steal to myself, the less time I would be forced into conversation, loud laughter, music and awkward questions. I suppose these questions are inevitable when friends and family are concerned. But my answers were odd, in the sense that NO ONE had ever heard of this thing called benzodiazepine withdrawal. And one question led to another, and to another, and to another, until I essentially became a teacher/victim in progress. I DID NOT WANT to talk this much, so I tried to be as succinct as possible. I also DID NOT WANT to appear to be needy, as it would take the attention away from the joy of the holidays and direct it towards pitiful me.

On the 27th, again the 4th day of the cutting cycle, I wake up to the world's worst stiff neck in the history of mankind, well beyond belief. All of the tendons in my neck feel like iron rods. They are very painful. They simply will not loosen up. They are visibly stiff, jutting from my neck. I can barely turn my head. My neck hurts; it feels like someone has the ends of the tendons fastened down to a turning device and is slowly tightening the tension. Jesus this hurts. It's like my neck is on "the rack". I have read about this on the board, but Christ, I didn't expect it to hit me, much less be this bad. Hyperacusis, anxiety, tinnitus, metal band around my head, adrenaline rushes, the "flu", impaired cognition and memory, and now my neck.

As I write this, I am corresponding with a current member of benzo.org.uk on multiple occasions throughout the day who has such severe neck pain and rigidity, as well as severe abdominal pain that she has now hinted at "giving up", which in her case means "reinstating". If I have any clue she meant suicide, I would call her and get her to a professional. Many sufferers feel this way. They feel that it just isn't worth the constant battle, so they will just take a little more poison than they are on and feel better. Well, they are probably correct (unless they are "in tolerance") for the short term. But in the not too distant future, symptoms would return and they would need more poison and find themselves right back where they started, only worse. In almost every case, this produces a much more horrific withdrawal, and one increases the probability of a protracted withdrawal, going on for years, for an as yet undetermined length of time. Tolerance withdrawal is exponentially worse than my experience: peak symptoms all the time, never a valley, always peaks. Unending suffering. At some point after the last dose, healing begins, but the prognosis is for a longer period of suffering than those not in tolerance withdrawal.

Throughout the day, I experience sharp pains in my neck (not my students, hahaha) that jab me here and there. I also notice that when I press 2 tendons in particular (on my right side), my tinnitus, which has elevated again, gets higher in pitch, as though I am playing a stringed instrument. This simultaneously intrigues and frightens me. There is an apparent relationship between my tinnitus and my muscular/tendon/ligament rigidity. That makes me happy, because I feel I have *some control over something.*
But the big picture is that I have yet another thing wrong with me. Another one. This isn't going to kill me, I know. I've read about this as being a very common symptom. Something is killing

my neck. I learn how to deal with this one, though "dealing with it" only helps a bit. Over time, I learn that ice packs after dinner throughout the evening and a little heat in the morning work best. I apply ice every night for months. The constant tugging on my muscles, tendons and ligaments are producing swelling, and the ice packs seem to help. Maybe they just numb everything. I'm not sure, but as it appears to lessen the pain, I stick with it.

I understand why this is happening in general. It's all about the nature of addiction. With each tiny cut, the addict's body, *my* body, gets really angry, and punishes me. This is a physiological reaction, plain and simple.

> *My God, now I understand why I can't make big cuts and make them more quickly. Oh, my God, I can't imagine any other way.*

I also begin the pattern of alternating Tuesday afternoons after school between acupuncture and a special chiropractor in a nearby city who also does acupressure massage. He is stunned at the condition of my jaw joint below my ears (temporo-mandibular joint). A past bodybuilder who has treated many boxers in his career, he has never felt such tightness here. He applies electric stimulation to my neck to try to loosen everything up, with very slow but steady progress over the next 5 months. When he massages this joint and applies pressure, the sound quality of my tinnitus changes, and again the pitch becomes higher with pressure. No one understands this, except Dr. Gary. He says he has seen similar types of tinnitus before with boxers. He believes that over time he will be able to either eliminate or substantially reduce the tinnitus. When I explain the withdrawal issue to him, he is right on board. My muscles are in a state of revolt, one of the many paradoxical results of benzo withdrawal. The very same benefits that these drugs have initially, such as muscle relaxation, twist around 180 degrees so that the drug/poison is now *causing the opposite effect*. And it won't let go easily. My neck muscles feel like there are machines on each end pulling in opposite directions. I am definitely on *the rack*.

Every time I leave Dr. Gary, the volume of my tinnitus is down a small amount, but my hyperacusis is up. I wish I understood this. Very little of it makes sense. Every time I find some aspect of this experience that makes sense, no matter how small or seemingly insignificant, I feel psychologically better. Even things that I do not understand at all that are somewhat predictable, such as the effect of massage on my jaw joint, are positive. I know what to expect. The uncertainty of this "ride" is quite an experience, especially for people like me who are logical by nature. It defies our need to find order wherever possible.

Another month ends.
All targets met.
All systems working.
All customers satisfied.
All staff eagerly enthusiastic.
All pigs fed and ready to fly.

-Anonymous

Chapter 21: January

January, February and March were clearly the 3 most difficult months, particularly given the trauma marching my way, steadily, beat by beat, in late January. March was also brutal, for it brought with it an old symptom with a renewed vitality and regularity: vertigo. I was again wearing down as a result of the constant assault from the unknown; a new symptom every week or so piled on. This was a repeated sequence. Beaten down, down, down, somehow lifted up, repeat.

In early January, I am in my bedroom as usual, door closed, light out as usual and on-line as always.

I hear people in the house. Who is in my house? There are people here somewhere! I know Maddie and I have not been close lately, but she would never have people over without telling me. Maybe they just stopped over and came in the front door without me hearing them. Given the layout of my house, this is a reasonable hypothesis. But I am wondering why they are here and why so many. Sounds like at least a half-dozen guests, more like a dozen or so, off in a distance. I

111

open the door, call for Maddie, and close it while I wait.
Maddie opens my door and says, "Yes?"

S: *Who is here?*
M: *Here? (yes) In the House? (yes) No one but us.*
S: *What? Is the TV on loud?*
M: *No.*
S: *That's weird. Sorry.*

I return to my world at benzo.org.uk. At this point in time, I am mostly responding to the needs of others, trying my best to help them, especially newcomers. I remember what it was like to stumble upon this site, benzo.org.uk. I was confused and frightened at first, as are many of the "newbies".

There are those people again. I hear them clearly, though I cannot discern even one word. I creep over to the door and crack it open. No change in the sound. That was a clue unrecognized. I am afraid to go out there, to leave the safety of my sick room, but I do, growing ever annoyed at these people for being in my house and at Maddie for apparently lying to me. This makes no sense now, but it was perfectly logical then. I go from room to room. No one there. I stop for about 2 minutes in the pantry and just listen. Maybe the sound is outside. There it is again. People talking! Lots of them! I open the door to the back, screened-in porch. Nothing. I wait. There it is again! It's exactly the same volume wherever I go.

I scurry back to my bedroom, like a little scared mouse running for cover. I am thinking this through. It takes me a couple of days worth of searching around the house and property to grudgingly come to the only reasonable conclusion. I am having auditory hallucinations. I'm certifiable. Me, Mr. logical, a complete, total, raving lunatic. I wonder to myself if it still "counts" as an hallucination if I recognize it as such. I have an internal debate about it. Finally, I conclude, who the hell cares and what's the difference.

About 1 week later, the phone is ringing in the kitchen and I know Maddie is out there. Maddie, please answer the phone. I yell it out. I think please answer the goddamn phone! Jesus! You are standing right there! Maddie opens the door to the bedroom.

M: Sam, the phone is not ringing.
S: Yes it is, honey...I just heard it.
M: I was standing right here. No ringing.

I am really frustrated about this. I heard the freaking phone. Clearly! It rang 7 or 8 times. Jesus, how can she say it wasn't ringing? But Maddie does not lie, and I know this. There is no reason for her to say this if it were not true. I conclude that there must be a crossed line somewhere and it is ringing in the line below my bedroom in the basement. I wait for it. There it is! I run out the bedroom door anxious to capture this beast of a ringing phone and down into the basement I go, over to the side below my bedroom. Nothing. I wait. Nothing. Crap.

Back in my bedroom a few minutes later, I hear the bloody phone ringing again. I drop to the floor, ear to the boards just outside my bedroom, where there is a little gap in the very old wood flooring. Not down there in the basement. Not in this room. I don't move. I hear it. Then it hits me. It's the same volume wherever I am. Another hallucination. My chin drops to my chest. I am mentally exhausted. Depleted. I am so tired of fighting this crap off. It never, ever goes away. Never. Now the phone is ringing in my head.. Jesus. Help. I need a break.

The only "break" I get is for a few hours or sometimes half a day as the result of having acupuncture. My tinnitus and anxiety dim for a short while. It really helps. Some control, though not much. Voices in the distance and the telephone ringing will continue for a while, about 2 months. I know they are not real, and, with significant effort, I learn to ignore them.

I continue with 2 mg. cuts in January on the 4th and 15th. The cut on the 15th is very hard. It brings me down to zero mg. at midday. I am happy to reach this milestone, but my angry body is not. It is very angry, angry as hell, really mad. Anxiety goes through the roof. Acupuncture doesn't help this time. I don't know how much more I can bear. My symptom list is growing and I can't take much more. Add to the list powerful facial pain and pain in my teeth on one entire side of my face.

Severe Anxiety
Moderate to Severe Tinnitus
Horrible Hyperacusis
Agoraphobia
Generalized fears
Metal band tightening around my head
Flu-like feelings
Rigid neck
Painful, swollen neck
Auditory hallucinations
Facial pain
Multiple tooth pain
Abdominal Adrenaline rushes
Impaired Memory
Impaired cognition

NOTE: For a thorough list of symptoms, go to appendix A. This list will hopefully scare the hell out of you.

I yearn for my old friend today. I don't see how I can go on. Where are you? Ah, there, close by. Whispering. Smiling gently.

I hear you. I know you can help me.

Friend: Yes, Sam, I can help you when the path stops.
Sam: I need you. Are you near?
Friend: I am near, Sam. But I cannot help you yet.
Sam: No? Please, dear friend, I can't take much more
of this. I need help. My energy is fading. I do not know
how I can continue on.
Friend: Your life force is still strong, Sam. You are stronger
than you think.
Sam: I don't feel strong, my friend. I just keep moving
forward somehow. I don't know how. One minute follows
another.
Friend: Yes, forward, Sam. Forward. Time is still there in
your forward path. You are free to move.
Sam: Still? But how?
Friend: Yes, Sam. Free to move. The path is not ended.
You will call for me soon but I will not answer. The path will
not yet be ended.

I am disappointed. Why can't I just end? I want to end. And then, just when it can't possibly get any worse, it does.

Life has got a habit of not standing hitched. You got to ride it like you find it. You got to change with it. If a day goes by that don't change some of your old notions for new ones, that is just about like trying to milk a dead cow.

- Woody Guthrie

Chapter 22: Sheeba

When Maddie and I moved into our home in August of 2002, a beautiful, lake home, we noticed that every day without fail, a black, long-haired dog with a wisp of white on her chest would take a stroll through the back of our property. Intent on her destination, a small horse farm to our north, she would barely acknowledge a hello. As time passed and she became more familiar with us, she would stop briefly, long enough for a pat on the head. Her visit would last longer and longer until she was spending more time at our home than anywhere else. Finally, in the spring of 2003, she sat on our back stoop and would not leave.

We did not know what to make of this. Where did she live? Was she just a wanderer? We inquired at the horse farm and found that they were also puzzled about her. She visited there every day. It seemed she was looking for food, and this suggested she was nomadic. There was evidence that she had a past hip problem as she walked with a slight tilting of her hips. She knew no commands. She was, above all else, a very gentle, sweet girl. She attached herself to Maddie in the spring and decided that she lived with us.

No one ever came looking for her. We put an ad in the local paper. Truth is, she adopted us. She simply chose to be with us, and we were delighted. Sheeba was her new name. She was a true companion dog who would follow us wherever we went when we were outside on our 3-acre parcel of land.

She was terrified of thunder, even distant thunder, and her legs would shake whenever she heard it, often before we did. She loved to be comforted during these times.

One of those dogs who seems to be able to sense emotional need in their master(s), she frequently found either one of us when we were struggling through this ordeal more than usual. During those times, she just sat beside us, or lay down beside us, frequently looking up. Or she would uncharacteristically lean against us while giving soft glances. It was only during those times of need that we all experience in our lives that Sheeba would, if your face was close to hers, give a tiny, soft, sweet little tip-of-the-tongue lick of your nose. Under most normal circumstances, she had her special places to be. On warm summer days, when not outside, she would inevitably find the cool Italian tiles in the kitchen. On cold winter days, she would lie down next to a radiator.

Though a slightly older dog, she was quite independent, and still continued her daily treks around the neighborhood. She was street-wise, in that she would actually look for cars when she decided to "hit the road" and go visiting. I watched her on several occasions as she changed sides of the road to accommodate an approaching car. Maddie and I made a conscious decision not to change her daily routine, as this had been her life, and her apparent road/car knowledge gave us peace of mind. Sheeba valued both the loving home environment and her personal freedom.

In late January, with my list of withdrawal symptoms growing and growing and the benzodiazepine in my body growing angrier at its slowly diminishing available supply of Ativan, I was in a terrible state of mind. By this time, I had considering quitting my teaching job on several occasions, only to have the grim reality of losing my house force me to stay. We were barely getting by at the time, since my new job paid substantially less than the previous one. Additionally, the health insurance benefit was almost non-existent at the new job, whereas in the previous position, like many others, I was grand-fathered and paid almost nothing for my insurance.

I was withdrawing further and further into my bedroom universe, rarely coming out save to eat and do life's essentials. I did not realize it at the time, but there was another symptom I was dealing with, one that typically creeps up slowly during benzo withdrawal, and one that places the victim in a surreal world, where nothing seems "real" and everything is somewhat distorted. I would not comprehend the existence of this symptom until well into my recovery. Known as derealisation, a sort of zombie-like existence prevails. All emotions are muted but negative. There is no true happiness; positive emotions are gone or severely muted. To my recollection, it is perceptually similar to the beginning stages of intoxication, except that *everything, every second of the day,* is permeated with a bad feeling, almost a sense of doom.

Sheeba quickly learned that if she walked towards either Maddie or me with a happy, wagging demeanor, turned suddenly and then left the room, it meant she had to go out. We were well trained. And it was almost like clockwork that she would do this early every evening, even though she spent most of her day outside either on our small country estate or visiting neighbors. Always, in about 20 minutes, she would return, sit on the large, dark rock barely above the earth's surface outside our back door and bark every minute or two until we welcomed her back into her home.

In the deep darkness of late January 2004 on a cloud-covered night, new moon or both (I can only recall how profound the darkness felt), Sheeba asked to go out unusually late. Dutifully, but with a sense of foreboding, I let her out. To this day, I do not know why I felt any more uneasy about this action than I did about everything else I did at this time of withdrawal, but I have no doubt that there was a different quality about it. I would never see Sheeba's beautiful, soft face alive again.

Forty-five minutes later, Maddie and I took turns calling for Sheeba, yelling her name into the void of the night every 5 or ten minutes. Something was wrong, and I knew it. I knew it as I let her out, but did not act on this intuition. Finally, we became so worried that we went out walking first, down the snow-lined country road outside our home in both directions, calling, whistling and praying inside. The snow banks were several feet high along the road. With each call for Sheeba, my ears buzzed and cracked inside my head. We listened intently for any response, perhaps a bark or whimper. Nothing. Blackness all around. Emptiness within and with the outcome of our search growing more likely by the minute, we went by car to much further destinations than Sheeba had, to our knowledge, ever been. Nothing. We returned home. We called and called. We walked to the end of our driveway and stood silently, listening. Maybe she was hurt and would call for us. Maybe she was at someone's house, inside, spending the night.

Finally, at about 2:00 a.m., we abandoned the search till morning, a work day. Maddie tried her best to reassure herself and me.

As I lie down in bed, she closes the door and says, "Everything will be okay; Sheeba will come back in the morning." My response is a loud, stern statement of knowing, somehow knowing. "She's dead."

I have a dream, a rare dream. Or do I? Very short, I hear in the distance, 3 soft, painful yelps. I sit bolt upright. My heart is pounding. Is she hurt? Is she out side by the door? I jump up and go to the door. The silence pierces the cold, black, damp air. She is not there. I check all of the doors. Nothing. I open the doors and listen. I call her name. I listen. The darkness is laughing at me. I go back to bed. I listen and listen. A dream. It must have been a dream………no, a nightmare. Oh, God, I hope it was a dream. I fear what the morning will bring.

Maddie leaves the house a little earlier than usual, planning to look more thoroughly in the growing light. I am standing at the kitchen counter, sipping tea. Seconds later, she appears at the door. Our eyes meet. They become one. Instantly, I know that she has found Sheeba. I turn my body to her and say her name softly, almost inaudibly, pitifully. "Maddie? Is it Sheeba?" Maddie is still in shock. Her mouth is slightly open. Her mouth is quivering. She nods her head. I pause for a few seconds. Then I ask, "Is she dead?", praying for the answer that I know will not come. Instantly, she begins sobbing and says, "Yes." As loud as I have ever screamed, the word, "NO!" bursts from the depth of my being. As I scream, electric shocks curse through the entire left side of my body, from my head to my toes, as though I am being electrocuted. They continue for about 10 seconds. I am paralyzed. Then they pass. Maddie is in my arms, sobbing. I cannot see; the tears are too thick. We are a pathetic mass of profound, traumatic grief.

An eternity passes.

Maddie says, "Sam, we have to go get her." I scream, "NO, NO, NO, NO, NO! I can't do it, Maddie! I can't do it!" My ears rumble and buzz loudly with each word.

    We stumble outside, clinging together, bending over in agony as we get closer to Sheeba. I can barely see her. She is at the end of the driveway, on the right side, just over the edge of the snow bank. Her black body stands out against the soft, glistening white snow. I can't go closer. Over and over I sob, "I can't do it. I can't do it."

    "She has to go into the barn, Sam. She will be safe there." She is crying deeply. I have never seen her like this. "Maddie, I can't look at her. I CAN NOT. I don't want to look at her dead." Yet, I know I have to do this. I am physically the correct choice. "Get me a sheet. I can cover her."

    As I approach her, cars are passing by. I am yelling, sobbing, "God, no! God, no!" I get close trying not to look. I catch a glimpse of her eyes, slightly rolled up into her head. Her tongue is out of her mouth a little, motionless. I cover her with the sheet and force part of the sheet under her through the snow. I am on my knees sobbing. I lift her up, carry her to the barn, and place her gently there, on a bed of hay. She is heavy. She is dead.

Both Maddie and I feel like we can die. In fact, we both want to die. We cannot find anything good to live for. Maddie is now clinically depressed. I am in the clutches of a deep-clawed demon. Sheeba is dead.

I call and call for friendship to bear fruit, finally. I want my path to end, desperately. I no longer want to be free to move. Where is a good friend when you need her? Sadness surrounds me everywhere. I am numb, yet suffering deep pain. Withdrawal symptoms all are worse than ever. I just want to die. Let me die, please.

Exactly one week later, alone in my classroom, I am thinking of Sheeba. My cell phone rings, but as I do not recognize the number, I do not answer it. A minute later, it rings again. Same number; I do not answer it. It rings yet a third time. Enough. I pick it up to silence; no one is there. About a minute after I hang up, there is a message. This is odd, I think. I retrieve the message. It is only one word long. I play it over and over in disbelief. How can this be? I call the number to find that it is the racquetball club that I played at briefly a year earlier. I inquire about the message. They do not have an automated message capability. The message is still with me, a soft, somewhat mechanical female voice. One word, a message that I kept for over a year after Sheeba's death. One simple word.

"Goodbye."

Sheeba was with us during the darkest times. I told her I loved her frequently. She was a vital part of our lives for about 20 months. And while she left when I was in need, she left perhaps knowing, somehow sensing things only the way dogs can, that I was finally on the road to better health. Indeed, in a month or so, after the electric shocks subsided and disappeared, there would be small signs of returning health.

I wonder about that message. Logical in thought and practical in behavior, I still wonder. Maybe there are things we do not understand, forces at work beyond our grasp, marvelous little joyful mysteries all around us as we take this voyage through the unknown that we call life. Are angels real? Can they come to us disguised as animals? Perhaps each one of us is softly yet firmly nestled in the arms of an angel during the most difficult times of our lives. I played that message hundreds of times, listening intently for some clue, *anything* to help solve this puzzle. The mystery of it all managed to breathe life back into me, to free the path forward again. Maybe it really was Sheeba saying goodbye. Maybe, just maybe, it was. Maybe Sheeba knew this was the only way I would be able to make it, regularly wondering about the mystery of that one-word message from nowhere, from oblivion. Perhaps it was Sheeba who kept two old friends apart.

"Goodbye, Sheeba."

All things arise,
Suffer change,
And pass away.

This is their nature,

When you know this,
Nothing perturbs you,
Nothing hurts you.

You become still.

It is easy.

--Ashtavakra Gita 11:1 (Hindu)

Chapter 23: February

During the month of February, many new symptoms appeared.
Thus far, I had accumulated a fairly long list:

Severe Anxiety
Moderate to Severe Tinnitus
Horrible Hyperacusis
Agoraphobia
Generalized fears
Metal band tightening around my head
Flu-like feelings
Rigid neck
Painful, swollen neck

Auditory hallucinations
Facial pain
Multiple tooth pain
Adrenaline rushes
Impaired memory and cognition
Electric shocks
derealization

The electric shocks lasted only about 3 weeks, thankfully. At first a few times a day, then twice, then only once, slowly diminishing in intensity, they were finally gone. If I were to judge all my symptoms in isolation, without considering longevity or severity, these electric shocks, somehow arising on their own from my head to my toe directionally, would top the list. It isn't the most fun to exist in a state of expectation when that expectation involves a feeling of electrocution. They weren't tiny zaps; they were strong jolts that made me feel like I had my finger in an electric socket. Added to my changing list in February were:

A constant metal taste in my mouth
Anal cramping
Fasciculations: a small, local, involuntary muscle contraction (twitching) visible under the skin
Formications: sensation of small crawling insects on the skin
Pretend tooth infections
Inner vibrations

Looking back, I cannot fathom how I was able to tolerate this manner of existence every day. I can say without a doubt that I had placed my hope in the hands of the beautiful administrators, moderators and members at benzo.org.uk. They didn't let me down. I placed my life in the hands of God. It's still there, just as it has always been and always will be.

The good news is that while these symptoms were added, several were in the process of disappearing or had disappeared during this month. Gone or going were both the constant flu-like feeling and metal banding around the head. Auditory hallucinations were almost done by the month's end. The big three, anxiety, tinnitus and hyperacusis were ever-present. Anxiety fluctuated in severity with the wind, from moderate to severe. Tinnitus varied from reasonably low, say a 3-4 on a scale of 10, to severe, an 8. Once in a blue moon, I had no tinnitus upon awakening for a brief period of time, minutes at best. I am certain that there were other symptoms that I do not recall at the present time, but this isn't significant.

On February 12, tinnitus comes roaring so loudly (10) as I am leaving school, that I cannot hear people speaking in a normal tone of voice at all. Imagine a sound in your head so loud that you can hear nothing else, a sound that you cannot stop, and a sound that sounds like a combination of a jet engine plus a generator plus bacon frying. Nothing I can do changes this sound. All the little tricks that I have learned to alter the pitch fail.

Upon my arrival home at about 4:30 p.m., I grab a flexible ice pack, go into my bedroom, close the door, light out, and lay in bed for 6 hours before the sound lessens. Not much, but enough to return to some semblance of sanity. I respond to no one during this time, eyes closed. I keep repeating in my head, "This will pass, this will, pass, this will pass....." I never thought I would be thankful for a "normal" tinnitus volume (6), but on that night it was the difference between standing next to Niagara Falls and a normal rain shower. Finally, it lowers a little, and I sleep.

Sometime between sleep and blaring tinnitus, I wonder how long I will have to persevere. I wonder why I can't die when I want to. It seems like an eternity since this began, even though it has been only 6 months since tinnitus first appeared, a harbinger of a living hell changing from bad to worse. Yet it has been 16 months since my life changed completely, the result of that fateful "meeting" in the fall of 2002. More than this, it seems like I am bearing a barrage of symptoms the depth of which I cannot even now believe. No one

else can possibly understand this, except the folks at benzo.org.uk.
This experience is "normal" there. They understand.

To the reader: If you are interested in what it is like to have
tinnitus, there are several tinnitus simulator sites on the internet at
this writing. Use your search engine, and then play the simulator
for as long as you can stand it in earphones........I bet you won't last
long.

The Feb. 12 tinnitus attack from hell would be, praise to God, the very last *severe* tinnitus I would experience. When I wake the next morning, it is down to a 4. I wish to be clear that 4 is no picnic. There is still a damn noise in my head and it still won't go away. But the horrible, unthinkable levels would never return.

On Feb. 11, I had made a cut from 15 mg. Valium (diazepam) per day to 14 mg. I was cutting both my evening and morning dose equally, half a milligram each. All sorts of fears were released as a result of my Feb. 12 response, only 1 day later. All of my other symptoms elevated after this cut for about 7 days. The old pattern was gone out the door. This was different. The moderators and administrators at benzo.org.uk were, as always, right. Unpredictability was the rule.

On Feb. 22, I make another 1 mg. cut to 13 mg. Magically, miraculously, unbelievably, my body does not respond. My body does not respond. It simply does not respond. I keep waiting for the inevitable, but something has changed. My body does not respond. Not even 1 symptom flares to severe levels. After about a week, I begin to have forbidden thoughts!

Maybe I am getting better! Maybe we have passed a key
point in time! Shhhhhhhhhh! Don't think it! Don't tell
anyone! Keep it a secret! Maybe I am on the road to
recovery! Shhhhhhhhhh! I can't think it. Something will
happen and everything will come back. Don't think it. Stop
it!

I am so excited by this prospect, that I make a key decision. The final act in a process of surrender to the forces of the universe, I completely release myself, willfully, from worrying about my future. I am praying more than I ever have, and I am not worried any more. Prayer seems to be helping me a great deal as I decide to willingly place my life in the hands of God. Psychologically and spiritually, I am lifted up. This is a remarkable development. After months of complete self-absorption, with a severe hypochondriac's level of self-concern, micromanaging every minute of every day, I was able to just let go, to finally fully resign as general manger of the universe. I decide to make very small cuts the rest of the way. I would make only .5 mg cuts on a weekly basis. In doing so, I was committing myself to at least 26 more weeks of tapering, 6 months more of the same. However, I was now able to free myself from the grip of time. No more pushing the envelope. Time disappeared. This is, in and of itself, a magical experience. I was just going to let the universe and the God of my universe proceed as planned. What could I do anyway? A friend tells me, "If you want to make God laugh, tell her what your plans are." I get it. Completely. I'm not in charge. Not at all! And so it was.

To this day, I spend time during quiet moments pondering my existence absent the concept of time. This would be the ultimate surrender, a surrender to a loving and omniscient God.

> *The ancient masters were profound and stable.*
> *Their wisdom was unfathomable.*
> *There is no way to describe it;*
> *All we can describe is their appearance.*
>
> *They were careful*
> *As someone crossing an iced-over stream.*
> *Alert as a warrior in enemy territory.*
> *Courteous as a guest.*

Fluid as melting ice.
Shapeable as a block of wood.
Receptive as a valley.
Clear as a glass of water.

Do you have the patience to wait
Until your mud settles and the water is clear?
Can you remain unmoving
Till the right action rises by itself?

The Master doesn't seek fulfillment.
Not seeking, not expecting,
He is present, and can welcome all things.

Lao-tzu

Reminds me of my safari in Africa. Somebody forgot the corkscrew and for several days we had to live on nothing but food and water.

- W. C. Fields

Chapter 24: Self-Care

Ever since the appearance of hyperacusis, my diet changed out of necessity. Then, after finding benzo.org.uk, I changed what I ate even further. This change was based on fear and the result of taking every bit of advice that the forum gave me along with the advice of Dr. Heather Ashton via her "How to Withdraw" Manual.

When hyperacusis first appeared it was not severe, yet within a week, it became obvious that I could no longer consume any food that was the least bit crunchy. When I did, the sound was amplified ten-fold! The volume was so high that it was painful. Can you imagine a crunching noise so loud that it actually causes pain or discomfort so loud that it might as well be pain, all coming from inside your head?

As a champion salty-snack food eater, that meant no more chips of any variety, no nuts, no crunchy fruits like apples, and no raw vegetables like carrots and celery. I couldn't eat salads, either. Vegetables can be cooked, and so can apples for that matter. But poor me could have no more chips, peanuts, almonds, etc.

The big change was chips: regular, wavy, garlic, cheesy, corn chips, potato chips, etc. Unfortunately, these snacks had been a big part of my diet. Even celery in salads like tuna salad and chicken salad was a problem. If I chose to eat either of those, I would have to search around for the pieces of celery and chew them so carefully and slowly that it would take me forever to eat. None of these changes were bad! I knew at the time that my weight would begin to change.

The administrators and moderators at the forum also advised me, as Ashton's work suggests, to lower my carbohydrate intake, lower my sugar intake and avoid caffeine and alcohol. I internalized this advice. In fact, until June, 2004, I had NO sugar in my diet other than what can be found in an orange, watermelon or other soft fruit, NO caffeine, NO alcohol, and a VERY low carbohydrate intake. The caffeine and sugar was not a major issue, as I did not typically take in caffeine or sugar other than in the form of chocolate. So, no more chocolate, period. None. No sugar. No caffeine. None. Also, I had a very low carb intake, as I limited myself to 1 slice of bread per day and no packaged, processed foods. Anything with a carb count over 9 was too high. Period. This was a big change, as I was also a champion sandwich man. Finally, I took no alcohol, which was very easy for me as I rarely consumed alcohol anyway. Alcohol, it seems, operates on the same receptors as benzodiazepines. No thanks. I don't need any more trouble.

The bottom line was that I was maintaining a healthier diet than I ever had in my life, except for the absence of salads and other crunchy, healthy food. But I did have cooked down greens to compensate for this. The result? By June 1rst, I was 70 pounds lighter, and fast approaching my ideal weight. It's amazing what someone can accomplish when they live every day in fear.

It was difficult for me to understand how other victims on the forum would continue to take alcohol and/or caffeine. Both clearly cause an increase in symptoms. That was the last thing I wanted. I concluded that they were either not suffering so badly or they were addicted to those other substances as well.

I remember clearly an "incident" early on in my withdrawal phase, in early September, just before hyperacusis hit. I was in the faculty room at my new school. Now, faculty rooms in many schools are known to be places where people bring snacks to share, for general faculty consumption. This was one of those faculty rooms. It was morning, and I did not have any symptom other than strong anxiety at this point in this day. There were chocolate bars for sale as a fundraiser for the child of a faculty member. I took one, put my dollar in the provided envelope and promptly ate the chocolate bar. No less than 15 minutes later, tinnitus appeared, and it was fairly loud.

I remember wondering if there was a connection between either the sugar or the chocolate in the bar and the onset of tinnitus. Later, after I made the discovery of benzodiazepine addiction, it all made sense. My conclusion was simple: stay away from both! I did, however, believe (and still do today) that caffeine was the culprit. As a stimulant, the power of caffeine is underrated in my opinion, and its effect on someone in withdrawal, where the nervous system is already severely compromised, is considerable.

Hyperacusis had other effects on my behavior. I could not even dream of going out to eat at a restaurant, as the sound of many people in combination with plates and silverware crashing into one another would cause me to bolt to the freedom of outdoors. I could not eat lunch in the school cafeteria. I could not eat with other people, period. This meant never having guests, never visiting someone for a meal, and most importantly, always eating alone.

Even when Maddie and I would dine alone at home, two plates would hit together, or a fork would hit a plate or a spoon would smash against a glass or some great sound would happen and cause me pain, discomfort and upset. If Maddie committed the offense, I would glare at her in disbelief that she would be so inconsiderate. In truth, with normal hearing, it would be nothing, absolutely nothing. At the time, however, I did not understand this. And with every loud, booming, popping, crackling noise, my anxiety would skyrocket *instantly*.

So, most of the time, I ate alone, and that was perfectly fine with me.

Clean-up was a problem. I could not be in the vicinity if someone cleaning up. I would either become upset at the lack of consideration, bear the noise and grimace while feeling my anxiety shoot up to the roof, or suddenly and quickly leave the room.

On the other hand, clean-up was best left to me, though I hated it. It would take me forever, as every single movement with dishes, glasses and silverware was in slow motion and made with such enormous care that it looks really absurd to anyone who would happen to watch. Plate on top of plate, each piece of silverware put away carefully and properly, and one glass at a time were all carefully laid to rest with the skill of the universe's best surgeon. It was as though I was trying not to set off a bomb. And if something were to slip or if I were careless and miscalculated a placement, BOOM, and I would curse myself violently in whisper form.

The end result of all of my symptoms, but perhaps mostly tinnitus, is that I withdrew into the singular world of me. I appeared to be unfriendly to those who did not know me, which was almost all of my new colleagues. My new students must have wondered what manner of critter was suddenly teaching them mathematics. Yet, they did, for the most part, take very good care of me, making almost every possible attempt to stay unusually quiet.

Magnesium Citrate

During withdrawal, it is best to avoid supplements. Many of these products, in fact most of them, tend to make things worse. Chinese herbs, poorly controlled, are impure and can send symptoms through the roof.

The B vitamins are known to cause serious responses, too. Some antibiotics are extremely bad, and severely ratchet up symptoms. Both Benzo.org.uk and The Benzo Book detail this information.

There are those quick to take advantage of benzo sufferers and offer them cures right and left. It is easy to fall prey to these scoundrels.

In the course of my withdrawal process, I found that one thing was helpful to me, and I want to make it clear that it does not appear to help everyone in withdrawal. Some people respond poorly to it, or seem to, given the unpredictable course of symptoms. Some people cannot make use of it because they struggle with diarrhea.

Elemental magnesium citrate in powdered form was helpful to me in moderating the tense, tightly wound muscles in my body, particularly my neck. Most of us in the western world are deficient in magnesium, which is critical to the healthy functioning of our muscles and nerves. Among many other benefits, it can also help keep our blood pressure low.

It is my opinion that magnesium citrate taken in powered form in hot water can have a small but not insignificant positive impact during withdrawal. It is not a cure, not by a long shot. But it can help *some* people.

The very best product out there is unquestionably Peter Gilham's "Natural Calm". I recall the very first time I tried it. About 30 minutes before bed, my neck was so very tight and painful. The pain was constant and my neck felt somehow attached incorrectly to my body. I drank the hot magnesium tea. It warmed me, of course. But about 15 minutes after I finished the very last drop, I heard and felt a pop or crack in my neck. And then another, and a third snap. Maddie actually heard one of the pops. My neck vertebrae were actually self-adjusting, as though someone was releasing the machine that was pulling my neck muscles so tightly. I was surprised and startled a bit at the first pop. It offered me some relief from the tightness.

To this day, I take this product nearly every day. However, always be careful when taking any supplement in withdrawal. Most of the time they don't help at all or make things worse.

There is no good arguing with the inevitable. The only available argument with an east wind is to put on your overcoat.

-James Russell Lowell

Chapter 25: The Winds of March II

And so, on March 2, I begin the process of cutting .5 mg. of poison weekly, alternating between my evening dose and my morning dose. Six months and counting! After having no reaction to the last 1mg. cut, I am very confident that the remainder of this ride will be steadier, more tolerable. On Saturday, March 6, hope gives way to reality once again.

Still quite symptomatic, I am sitting in the office of my chiropractor, having rescheduled a Tuesday appointment for a reason that has escaped my memory. I feel okay, but I am getting quite warm. I ask to turn down the TV, as it is too loud for me. No one objects. Suddenly the world turns visually sideways.

Oh crap, what is this? Focus, Sam. Blink, blink, blink. Focus.

But every time I blink, the distortion resets itself, moving counterclockwise, then clockwise, right, left, up, down all at the same time.

Okay, time to get out of here, go to the bathroom. I'm getting sick. Fast. I remember this. CRAP! It's BACK! Oh boy. Here we go again. I know this feeling.

The vertigo that I had experienced about 10 months earlier was back. I make my way to the bathroom by holding on to the walls with two hands, peeking out from behind closed eyes every few seconds. I sit in the bathroom; it's safer.

Here it comes. Oh boy. Get to the sink. I dry heave about 6 times. No breakfast. Back to the toilet bowel. Sitting, catching my breath. Felt like I wasn't ever going to breathe again. I'm ok. I'm ok. Jesus, I am sweating. I feel my shirt; it is completely soaked. Holy cow, that was fast. After 10 minutes or so, I go back to the waiting room, in case they call my name. The 2 people in there stare at me. My eyes are mostly closed, but I peek now and then. The world is still spinning. I am drenched and my hair is soaked. One of the patients asks me if I am okay. I say yes, thank you. The receptionist sticks her head out of the window and she, too, asks if I am okay. I provide assurances. She tells me it will be at least 10 more minutes. I am really, really hot. The room is still tilted. I can't focus. I tell her I'm going outside to cool off. I find my way by touch, with an occasional peek, outside. It's a little better with my eyes closed. Looking at the world makes things worse. As I cool off, the visual world resets and stays put. Whew. Relief.

My chiropractor is hesitant to treat me. I assure him that this is probably a typical withdrawal symptom, even though I am not positive myself. He understands and does his thing. He tells me that the musculature of my neck and jaw is softening a little. I am happy to hear this, and it confirms my suspicions. There are little signs that things are getting better, and this is one of them. My tinnitus has not flared for 3 weeks. And until today, no new symptoms have appeared for a couple of weeks. All positive indicators.

As of this day, I am on March break, a 1-week vacation from school. I agree to take a 2-hour trip to see my youngest daughter and son-in-law. It is the first time I have ventured far from home for about 18 months.

When I arrive at Jamie's house, I immediately feel uncomfortable. I do not know why, but my anxiety is elevating. I am feeling fearful. There are dogs barking on both sides of the house. It is upsetting to me and loud to me. I can't sleep with 2 dogs barking in my ears. The baby, my beautiful granddaughter, isn't feeling well, and is whining and crying at times. Oh no, no, no, no. Please stop. I realize I shouldn't have attempted this trip. I can't stand it longer than 2 days and we leave 3 days early. On the way home, Maddie breaks down. She misses normalcy. I have worn her down and out. She is depleted. It is all my fault. I have intense feelings of guilt. As we drive, every time the front wheels hit the joint on the highway, it sounds like a bomb. All I want is the safety of my bedroom. I am a failure. I have ruined Maddie's life. I am bad. I wonder if Maddie will leave me. I deserve it.

On March 15, I return to school on a day of a cut, which is now every Monday. I am down to 11.5 mg., more than half-way home in terms of dosage. On Tuesday, vertigo attacks start coming fast and furious, nearly every day for about 3 weeks. Sometimes, they are only minor, with a small amount of disorientation. Other times, I am forced to walk, with my eyes closed lest I vomit on the spot, to the school nurse's office to lie down in the dark, eyes closed. This happens about 5 times in all, and each time a colleague must cover my class for me. In two of the five instances, I must crawl on my hands and knees the final 30 feet or so to the nurse's office. Fortunately, I have already warned the nurse that anything was possible in withdrawal, and not to be surprised. She was incredibly cooperative and understanding, and took the time to read some paperwork I had prepared for her from benzo.org.uk. I recall a day when my blood pressure fluctuated wildly in her office: 178/92 and then 3 minutes later 124/70, another classic benzo symptom. Before

I leave the classroom the first time, I am somehow able to tell the children that I am experiencing some dizziness, the result of a medication I am taking. I describe vertigo. It satisfies them. I sleep in the nurses office for about 60-90 minutes each time.

On Saturday, March 27, I experience a strong vertigo attack while driving. The onset is fast. At first I cannot read a road sign up ahead. Then the world twists, and I quickly exit the road, barely off to the side, turn off the car, shut my eyes and manage to fall off quickly. I call Maddie on my cell just as I am nodding off, so that she does not worry. When I awake, 3 ½ hours have passed, and I am stunned. The drive home is slow and cautious, as this time, there are some remnants of the episode that leave me feeling odd.

The day after this roadside event, my anxiety drops significantly to a level I haven't felt in a long, long time. I am completely baffled by this chain of events, but again I am hopeful. Anxiety flavors everything else.

I can't believe how lucky I am on this day.

Only industrial society has put a value on time, and we realize that time is insignificant because our own lifetime in this world is but a blink of the eye. And when you have that knowledge, that life is beautiful and you can enjoy it rather than worry about it, then you can even accept death just as you accept birth as part of the total sacred loop of life.

- Russell Means

Chapter 26: Windows and Recovery

On April 1, I experience what is known in benzo circles as a window, a temporary period of time during which one or more symptoms disappear completely or nearly completely. I wake up to a complete absence of anxiety. I simply cannot believe it. No more vertigo either. For 6 consecutive days, I have absolutely no anxiety. I am overjoyed beyond comprehension. It is working. The slow, steady taper of Dr. Heather Ashton and Ray Nimmo is working! I am a different person. And I suddenly realize that most of my symptoms seem to be either gone or very, very low. When did this happen? I cannot pinpoint the time. Everything is a blur: My remaining symptoms are:

Moderate Tinnitus
Moderate Hyperacusis
Low, diminishing Agoraphobia
Generalized fears are diminishing
Rigid neck is changing
Painful, swollen neck is changing

Wildly fluctuating blood pressure

While anxiety did return after that 6-day window, it will never again be severe. I am clearly on the road to recovery. I am a different person, and everyone notices. Rather than the strained look of constant anxiety on my face, it is replaced by a normal appearance or even a smile! It is unbelievable. There are several windows over the next months, and with each one, I am feeling better and better. Thank God for windows. Thank God for Ray Nimmo and his band of teachers and nurturers. Thank God for the camaraderie of all of those suffering at benzo.org.uk.

The road was not without its bumps, even as I am clearly healing. For example, on May 22, I write on my journal/calendar that my anxiety is gone for sure. Gone. Completely gone for over 3 weeks now. It only returns here and there for a few hours at a time. And on May 29, I recognize that, for the first time since it arrived, my hyperacusis has dropped significantly. Sometimes I can actually talk without any distortion in my head. Sounds are not bothering me so much anymore. The world is quieting down. Now and then, I hum a quiet tune. I miss that.

But then on May 30, I have a vertigo attack so horrific, so brutal, I am certain that I must be getting sick all over again. I wake up on this day feeling odd, and before I return from my morning trip to the bathroom, the world has turned upside-down, inside-out, is twisting, turning and completely unrecognizable.

I can barely crawl on all fours without falling. Then I cannot move at all. I crash into the side of the doorway headfirst. I cannot find the opening. I have no sense of where I am. None. Opening my eyes is useless; there is nothing to see but a bizarre, distorted unreality. Besides, if I open my eyes, I become powerfully nauseated. This is far worse than any vertigo I have ever imagined. Maddie happens to be up and sees me on the floor struggling to find my bedroom. I ask for a bucket. Nausea is fast approaching, despite closed eyes. I cannot consider a trip to the bathroom. She places it under my hanging head. While I am on all fours, I heave over and over. I almost pass out. I am once again drenched with perspiration. Maddie helps me crawl to the bed. I cannot move at all, flat on my back. Even the slightest movement causes me to feel like vomiting. The light is off, curtains drawn, as the light bothers me. I am hot. Then I am freezing. I cannot even move my eyeballs while my eyes are closed without feeling like vomiting. I assume this will last a couple of hours. It is 7:00 a.m. Sixteen hours later, at 11:00 p.m., I can open my eyes and focus on the curtains for a second, no more, or I get sick again. I sleep through the night. In the morning, I am physically weak, as though I have had a week-long flu. But I am free to move once again. I get up, having lost an entire day of my life to a manner of vertigo beyond comprehension. I wonder if there will be more; maybe I am not getting well after all.

This day, May 30, marks the final severe surge in my battle with benzodiazepine withdrawal. No more severe symptoms, ever. Even though I am still taking the poison, 6.5 mg. per day, the worst of it is over.

I continue tapering. By Mid-June, all of my symptoms are gone or nearly gone, even though I still have almost 5 months of tapering to go. Ashton has seen this before in her clinical studies. By utilizing a cross-over and a slow, steady taper, I am an example of the textbook manner of recovery, having lost nearly all of my symptoms by taper's end. I have often wondered why I got so lucky. After all, in Ashton's work, her patients were individuals who had NOT already attempted to taper and failed. Yet, somehow, I experienced an early loss of symptoms.

At some point in June, I receive an email from James, one of the administrators of benzo.org.uk. James was the one administrator with whom I connected best, although Ray, Yvonne and Jackie were also wonderful. All the mods and admins were, but those mentioned were those with whom I felt most comfortable. Logical, succinct, caring, steady and honest, James was ever patient with my attempts to find logical patterns in this experience.

In this email, I am asked to be a moderator for the site. I have gained sufficient knowledge, according to James, to be a moderator. He has also noticed my reassuring approach to the suffering of other members. And like James, I am steady, almost impossible to ruffle.

Privately, I am overwhelmed at this request. I have come full circle. I will now be able to be an official helper, one whose words can save a life. It is difficult to express how much a benzo sufferer looks to others for help, especially from someone with a moderator or administrator label. These people know a lot and have been through a lot. Their words were critical to my future, every step of the way. I trusted them far more than doctors, that is except for *my* doctor. I know that when I was at my lowest points, I would make a post and then read the answers over and over and over, dozens of times, looking for any shred of encouragement or good news. And all of the moderators and administrators and many of the members/victims at this site were busy caring for others, nurturing, sometimes getting tough when it was appropriate.

And now, I could be one of them. I was so very, very, pleased and I took this request to heart. I know from experience how important my words will be. I accept the "position" and for the next year, I will be able to repay this site for all they have done for me with my time. Now that I am re-entering life again, I am increasingly busy, but I am able to devote about 45 minutes per day, sometimes more (several hours), and sometimes less, to the place that saved my life: benzo.org.uk. I am thankful to have this opportunity.

Everything exists, somewhere and forever.

- Father Brian McHugh

Chapter 27: Freedom

On June 7, upon my awaking from a long Sunday night sleep for my final week of classes, I realize after yawning loudly that something is different. Very different. My own voice seems to be normal, and other sounds are only a wee bit louder than I think they ought to be. I start to hum, louder and louder, my voice cracking from normal morning voice syndrome! But no buzzing in my head whatsoever. And as I sit on the edge of my bed, I start to review my most recent symptoms and recognize that they are all gone. Nothing left but this ever-so-slight hyperacusis, and a level of tinnitus so low that it cannot be heard except in an nearly soundless environment. As far as I am concerned, it is gone. The reality of this is exhilarating. I am a happy husband, teacher, father and grandfather. I am me again, for the first time in a long time. I am so thankful to be alive, to exist once again in the world that I once knew ages ago. I will never take anything for granted again, especially my health.

Then on June 17, the final change is realized. Now 2 days after cutting to 5.5 mg. of Valium, I am feeling quite well.

Maddie and I are outside working on our 3-acre country property, a place where we both love to be. We are doing some hand trimming of our beautiful specimen trees and shrubs. We find ourselves trying to cut a branch that is too big for any of our hand tools. I say, "Hang on". As though nothing was ever wrong, I walk into the barn and retrieve our small, gas-powered chainsaw. I walk to the tree, check the oil and gas, and pull on the starter-rope several times. Maddie is watching in silence. Finally, the saw fires up, as loud as ever. I reach up and quickly slice through the 5-inch diameter branch. I cut off another smaller branch immediately. I shut off the saw, and as I do so, I am suddenly in full realization of what has just happened. I just used a chainsaw like nothing had ever been wrong, as though this thing called hyperacusis had never existed, a beast that I had thought might be with me for the rest of my life.

"Did you see what just happened, Maddie? Did you see what I just did?" Maddie was staring at me with eyes wide open and a wonderful smile on her face. She nodded her head. "I didn't even blink an eye! I used the chainsaw without even thinking about it! And it didn't bother me at all! Normal sound! Normal sound! Oh my God!"

I put the saw down on the ground and began to run around the property with my arms high in the air, yelling, "Thank you God, Thank you God", over and over. I had beaten benzodiazepine addiction, and I knew from experience, that there is nothing quite like it in human experience. I had never felt so proud of myself in my life.

Unfortunately, all the while that my hyperacusis was dimming, so was the hearing in my right ear. Shortly after the chainsaw event, it was gone again completely, and has not returned. Initially hopeful that it would somehow reappear, it has not and likely will not. I have learned subsequently that Ativan can cause permanent neural hearing loss. Honestly, I am so pleased to be well again, that I do not mind being deaf in one ear.

The next 3 months of my taper were uneventful. There was an occasional brief surge in anxiety, but it did not last long. Back at 7 mg., I decided that, as I was entering the lower doses, considered to be from 5 mg. on down to zero, I would extend the length of time in between cuts to approximately 10 days, just as an extra precaution. I did not want symptoms to return. In fact, many benzo victims do experience a significant upturn in the level of symptoms as they enter into the lower doses, as each cut begins to be an increased percentage of the current dose. I would be there soon enough.

Nothing changes for me. I am either lucky, or I am reaping the rewards of a strict approach to this taper and the benefits of the slow taper. Perhaps I am genetically predisposed to a quicker recovery than most. I suspect it is a combination of everything. My next to last cut is 50%, from 1 mg. to .5 mg. Still nothing happens. I am almost home, and I can taste the victory. There has never been a battle like this for me, and this victory is beyond description.

My taper ends with a 100% cut on October 2, 2004, approximately an 11-month experience including the discovery of benzodiazepine addiction, cross, and slow taper. My day of freedom is a day I shall never forget. I am tearful at frequent times throughout the day. Tears of joy. I am back to being me again, back as a player in this mystery of life. Only I am stronger, filled with a deeper, more thorough understanding of other people. I feel blessed to be alive. I feel more vibrant. I am going to reach for the stars in my life, never again waiting for things to happen. I promise to myself never to be shy about playing guitar or singing in public.

I am more cautious about the nature of other people as a result of the discovery of serial bullies, but I am still willing to stand up for what is right. I pledge to myself that if I ever find myself working for someone who is unethical again, I will not stay. More than ever, I want to be part of an ethical, caring, nurturing society. However, I do understand that there are times when one needs to be tough.

I now understand what it feels like to be depressed. Depression is no longer an abstract notion, nor is anxiety. I have felt these two things deeply and have learned from them. They are powerful, powerful phenomena. I can help people who are suffering merely through understanding. I get it. If only everyone could feel these two demons for a short while, in order to further their understanding of those that suffer from them. I have walked in the shoes of others, and while time will dim my memory, I will never forget.

There is an important clarification to make here. While my symptoms nearly "ended" before my taper was over, for the next year or so, I still got oddball, weird symptoms that lasted for a few hours or a day, always very low in intensity. I barely took notice of them. I was a fortunate soul. *But it is critical to report here that some people who taper off benzos still have severe symptoms after the last dose. It can go on for years.* No one knows why there is this vast variation, but it is real. Perhaps it is only our own distinct physiologies that cause this. We are all wired differently.

How many cares one loses when one
decides not to be something but to be
someone.

-Coco Chanel (1883-1971)

Chapter 28: Graduation

At the forum, this is a big day for everyone who finds there way to it, and for everyone else, for it breeds hope. Like a seed that bursts forth, every time another benzodiazepine addict reaches the day of freedom, more fertile hearts are born, infused with a growing hope that one day, it will be "my turn". Everyone posts a message of joy, congratulations, happiness, etc. I had participated in this rite of passage many times in the past, watching as those who came before me made their way to freedom. There is no bigger day at the forum. It is the culmination of months (11 months, almost a year, for me) of incredibly hard work, fighting the battle of a lifetime. We all look forward to this for others as well as ourselves.

There is an incredible camaraderie here, as friendships formed grow into a mutual respect for each other's humanity and strength. We have felt each other suffer, sometimes deeply. We have watched new friends disappear, wondering if they are still alive. We move from a stage of helplessness and fear to, by the time we graduate, a time when we focus on the needs of others. We have had some fun along the way, too, as we know the people on the other end of our computers share our goals: drug freedom and returning health. We have reached out to each other; we have lost sleep in worry for each other. We are like no other club in the world, a club that suffers together for months or years, typically without ever meeting one another. We all have lost lives and we want them back. Most of us feel the icy breath of death around us, as we battle against constant overpowering fears that can easily turn us into a babbling, helpless ball of complaints. Worse, the relentless daily struggle can make us impotent against the power of self-destruction. But most of all, we are drawn together by hope and by the day of freedom. Now, after watching dozens and dozens graduate before me, it is my turn. Finally, at last, it is my turn.

Early in my taper, I could not imagine this day. I did not have the typical understanding of time; it was a lost concept, typical in withdrawal. All we feel is the daily battering and a vague sense of the future being the same thing, day after day. It doesn't help when loved ones or friends deny the existence of our suffering or suggest that we just reinstate our drug use. THAT is hard to deal with. But I was blessed. All of my friends and almost all of my family understood my struggle and supported me all the way, especially my wife, father, stepmother and daughter. My colleagues were outstanding as well, and my students responded at a level that was astonishing.

So, on my day of freedom, I know what I will find at the forum. I can't wait. It is a Saturday, and a special day for another reason. When I open the site, there it is, a special thread just for everyone to say congratulations. They do it well, with wonderful words and great graphics. Post after post, they just keep coming. I am moved to tears many times over the course of the next 2 days, as the posts continue. I have chills of excitement several times. I am free. I am free to move. Free to move forward. My path is free again. I have not felt free for a long time.

It was about 9 years earlier, and in my first marriage, that I had first heard the words, "You are free to move". I had been in a deep meditation, after focusing my thoughts around some unusual events in my childhood that I cannot explain to this day. Loud and clear, as I eased toward a state of wakefulness, I heard the words as though they had been spoken by someone right there in the room.

"You are free to move."

147

At the time, I was startled and did not know what to make of these loud words. Now I think I know what these words meant, finally. They were meant to push me forward to a new life, one that would finally allow me to be, after suffering intensely, free to move, free to truly live life.

And so it was, that on my mother's day of birth, Oct. 2, that I entered a new phase of life. Having passed away 10 years earlier, my mother had an unswerving confidence in me, as has my father. So it is fitting, that on her birthday, I returned this deep belief in me with a gift to myself so profound, I have hope that the rest of my life will be richer by far.

Mrs. Kanyer,

I plan to go to The National Cemetary in Santa Fe on May 15th. (Sunday) Let me know if you want to go with me. Take care,

Linda

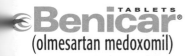
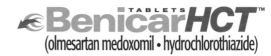

My theology, briefly, is that the universe was dictated but not signed.

- Christopher Morley

Chapter 29: The Big Picture

There are people in benzodiazepine withdrawal who find most days to be like my vertigo attack of May 30. Perhaps with different symptoms, they nevertheless cannot leave their bed due to a severe symptom or collection of symptoms. They are no less strong than I. Yet, their symptoms are simply worse, exponentially worse. Perhaps you know someone who acts oddly or seems always sick. If so, perhaps you now understand why. They may be fighting the benzo beast, one even bigger and more ghastly than the beast I defeated. Remember, recovery from this addiction isn't guaranteed. You can remain highly symptomatic well beyond the "last bit" of medication/poison.

But the unfortunate truth is that at this writing, benzodiazepines continue to be pushed by pharmaceutical companies. They continue to invent new versions.

Something must be done about it. In the UK and several provinces in Canada, any physician who administers/prescribes benzodiazepines for longer than 4 weeks is subject to serious professional sanctions.

What is taking so long in America? The facts of the matter have been clearly established, yet, benzos continue to be prescribed with little mention of the word "addictive". This is nothing short of criminal. Ahhhh. There's the answer. No one wants to be prosecuted. So, armed with the vast power of legions of lawyers employed by the pharmaceutical companies, benzos continue to

149

destroy lives and cause untold suffering. This is torture, plain and simple. And in some cases, it is murder.

Yet, there does not need to be vengeance or retribution, even though it may be well-deserved. We can control the future use of these medications easily. All it takes is a strong, interested congress, willing to simply set standards of use. One or two members of congress must step forward to start this process. I challenge all 435 members of the House and all 50 Senators to step up and do the right thing. Stop torture in our own country. Stop murder.

Pharmaceutical companies are staffed mainly by good, caring people who work hard to develop drugs to help people, to save lives. But there are those at or near the top that care about only one thing: getting rich. Make no mistake about it. These huge corporations are driven by money. Money is why they exist. Why can't this country have an FDA that isn't complicit? That's another book.

Healing is a matter of time, but it is
sometimes also a matter of opportunity.

Hippocrates

Chapter 30: On Doctors

There is a wide range of feelings within the benzo family, those
of us that have been and are addicted, relative to physicians, though
perhaps the emotion that comes through almost all positions is one
of feeling deeply betrayed. Now that I have come full circle and I
am well again, my perspective is somewhat different than the typical
perspective that I encountered at benzo.org.uk. No perspective is
necessarily right or wrong. But they are real, and they are all the
result of our own individual experience, which varies greatly.

I have been part of discussions with fellow victims in which we
plot our vengeance, perhaps through legal avenues or through silly
pranks. I have seen words of howling anger and bitterness. I have
heard words of forgiveness. I understand all of these words.

That we feel betrayed to some degree is likely not surprising.
After all, societies look to their "physicians" for health, whether
they are Shamans, acupuncturists, western doctors or priests. There
are many different categories of health, in both physical and mental
domains, and a variety of categories of "doctors". In the western
world, we mostly wait to be sick and then expect our doctors to treat
us with drugs to make us better. In other cultures, we expect spells
will ward off sickness, or we go to our physician when we are well
in order to stay well.

But when we get sick, we clearly extend the hand of trust to our physician(s) here in our western culture. We believe that our medical world is the best, and it likely is for the acutely ill. We know that doctors receive years of specialized education, training and practice. They are experts, and indeed, there are seemingly countless specialists in the medical world. Specialists are supposed to know a lot more about a lot less.

At the posting forum of benzo.org.uk, the original forum that literally saved my life, led me and sometimes pushed me through times of severe symptoms, I encountered hundreds of individual stories about how physicians approached benzo addiction and withdrawal. There were many times when I actually wanted the phone number of these physicians. They were stupid, arrogant, stubborn, childish people who not only created severe suffering, but refused to try to make things better even in the face of overwhelming evidence that they could, thereby extending and exacerbating suffering needlessly. I wanted to speak with these "physicians". These are the people from whom the arrogant, negative, uncaring, money-grubbing, ill-mannered, unethical physician stereotypes stem. They exist. In all occupations, there are poor examples. There is, no doubt, a continuum, ranging from superb to stinky, upon which we can place each and every physician we encounter. But the same can be said of teachers, lawyers, plumbers, etc. The big difference, of course, is the life and death issue inherent in the healing profession.

In my PTSD and benzo experience, there were 7 doctors/healers that were part of my journey: my general practitioner, ENT specialists (2), psychiatrist (one visit), therapist (clinical psychologist), acupuncturist and chiropractor.

Throughout my PTSD experience, my therapist, a past parent of 2 wonderful students of mine, was incredibly helpful. I had, over the years, seen the fruits of his work with some of my students. I had spoken with him on numerous occasions. He had helped my school through difficult times on more than one occasion involving tragedy. I had observed his approach with both of his children. His ability to articulate ideas and make profound insights into individuals and group dynamics was simply outstanding. When I realized I was ill and it wasn't a quickly passing phenomenon, I called him. He was booked, but he made room for me. I shall never forget that. He somehow shuffled his responsibilities as a Dean at the nearby University and created a time to see me. I knew that he would help me and indeed he did. His work with me, which inevitably involved making *me* think hard about something was the principle reason I recovered so quickly from PTSD. I am forever indebted to his kindness and skill.

Both my acupuncturist and chiropractor were also important to my ultimate wellness. The acupuncture work, along with essential oils, was astonishing to me. Some people, inclined to believe in only western medicine's approach to healing, have suggested that the acupuncture worked as it did, to lower my tinnitus and anxiety levels (temporarily), because I wanted it to or believed it would. However, to know me is to know that while I do have an open mind, I am essentially a skeptic by nature. I entered acupuncture and chiropractic care not having any presuppositions whatsoever. I was too sick to make projections. That I felt instantaneous relief from the tinnitus as a result of Carol *touching the rim of my ear* was a complete shock to me. I had never heard of essential oils before, and I did not now when to expect any change. Further, no subsequent visit produced effects quite as dramatic. If these changes were the result of a "placebo effect", why would they then diminish when I had become *more* hopeful? The acupressure and other work done by my chiropractor was clearly helpful in reducing the rigidity, swelling and pain in my neck and jaw. This was plain old hard work, with steady, small improvements each week. I could feel the slight changes in my jaw joint myself. Neck adjustments also produced two small but noticeable temporary changes; decreased tinnitus and increased hyperacusis. I have no explanation for this. I looked forward to both of these visits on alternating Tuesdays. They provided me with hope and some small, but vitally important measures of control over a process that had a life of its own.

I visited a psychiatrist only one time, as a consult for my general practitioner who felt dissatisfied with the generalized anxiety diagnosis. It didn't fit at all. The psychiatrist called my GP immediately and said that he had a definitive diagnosis: Post Traumatic Stress Disorder. I actually heard this conversation and was in full agreement with everything he said, as he listed the symptoms that matched. I was very happy to be properly diagnosed. Now I had something to sink my teeth into. I had *understanding.* That in itself was a small but nevertheless important consideration. No one likes not knowing what is wrong.

My ENT specialist was, in my opinion, a major problem. Actually, there were two of them in practice together. One was humble and worked hard to find out what was wrong. Unfortunately, he was not knowledgeable enough, otherwise he would have known that tinnitus can be caused by a sudden withdrawal from benzodiazepines. The other was arrogant and impatient, unwilling to have even a passing consideration of my thoughts. Remember, I actually asked if there was a relationship between my stoppage of Ativan and the tinnitus. Even a doctor without this knowledge who was genuinely a good doctor would have indicated uncertainty at this suggestion BUT then followed up with some brief investigation. He brushed my suggestion aside with a roll of the eyes as though it was foolhardy and I was a simpleminded fool. This is the manner of doctor that ought to be fed a diet rich in Xanax for a year or so.

Then there is my general practitioner, a damn good man. I know this man. He is one of those doctors who actually works hard to care for people day in, day out. He knows a lot more about eastern approaches to medicine than 99% of physicians, and for that I am thankful.

About 15 years ago, at approximately age 40, I was in significant and increasing pain in my neck and legs, mostly my legs. It was getting to the point that I had to physically lift my legs, one at a time, into first my underwear and then my pants. I had to walk like a tin soldier for about 30 minutes while my body slowly armed up. The pain was very unpleasant. Then, I would be basically okay for the day, with lingering pain. When I drove the car, a trip of more than 10 minutes or so caused very strong pain in the right leg, the one that applied steady pressure to the gas pedal. After exercising, the pain was genuinely severe. I would drive home after full-court basketball, sit down for 30 minutes or so at the computer or in front of the TV. Upon arising, it looked and felt like I was 100 years old. I had to crawl up the stairs to go to bed. Agony. My legs felt like lead and they did not want to work. They just plain hurt; not the joints, but the muscles.

I approached my GP about this one day with the suggestion that it might be fibromyalgia. My mother had fibromyalgia. I had not shared this information with him before. I had previously developed what now was clearly a foolish notion that I was just growing old a little faster than most people. After a thorough examination, he agreed. He also revealed that fibromyalgia was something he had more expertise in. He told me that I had a few options. One was a systemic approach advocated by western medicine that involved taking a steroid called prednisone. No way. My mother had been on it and the side effects were terrible. No moon face for me. There was another unusual option available, if I had an open mind. I could try sleeping on a mattress with magnets in the cover. I almost chuckled. Magnets?

He gave me the number of a lady who sold "magnetic mattresses" and would make one available for a free trial. Against my better judgment, fortunately, I called this lady sorcerer and set up the free trial. She advised me to try it for 1 – 2 full weeks and let her know what happened. Drink lots of water, too. Now that gave me a chuckle because I did not see any relationship. But what the heck? I started on a Monday night. By Thursday, I thought my legs were worse. On Sunday morning, I woke up and stood up with no pain. I was stunned. I tried lifting each leg. No pain, no stiffness. Gone. I felt like I did 15-20 years earlier. I was euphoric. Needless to say, to this day I still sleep on magnets, and they are slowly but surely being recognized as effective tools in pain management around the world.

So I had a history of valuing this doctor's opinion. He placed me on Ativan/Lorazepam because his training suggested that it would help my anxiety. It did. He did not know it would cause me to be

155

addicted in the time frame over which I took the drug. He did offer me warnings not to stay on too long. How long was "too long" in his understanding? I do not know. He also knew that I was typically thorough in my own research, but perhaps did not recognize that I was too sick to engage in that in this case, the only time in my life that I did not "study up" as I should have relative to a medication. On the other hand, I did read the little pamphlet that came with the medication, and it never referred to *addiction* as a possibility. The warning has subsequently changed, but it is still weak.

Can we really expect a general practitioner to have full knowledge of all of the thousands of medications that exist, with literally hundreds of new meds introduced each year? No way. And even if somehow they could create a time warp and accomplish this, the information they would discover is a product of the people who are trying to make money on their sale: pharmaceutical companies. Do they publish all of the information? Hell no. Time after time, we learn about hidden results, information withheld during the process of approval.

My doctor listened carefully to me when I approached him with new information. Many do not. My doctor supported me all the way, right to the end. My doctor took advantage of this circumstance to actually learn something. That by itself is, in my opinion, the critical mark of a good doctor. In fact, my doctor has asked me if I would be available to help any future patients of his that might be interested in a slow taper off of their benzodiazepine.

I was damn lucky to have such incredible support from so many good people, at beno.org.uk and my life in general. My doctor jumped on board with a process he had not seen before. My principal gave me lots of extra leeway. My friends and family didn't desert me. They trusted that I knew what I was doing during the slow taper. I trusted Ray Nimmo and his website. I trusted in God. I leaned on my wife very hard. Many couples cannot withstand this ordeal and divorce.

Life can only be understood backwards; but it must be lived forwards.

- Soren Kierkegaard

Chapter 31: Life Isn't Supposed to be Easy!

I shall never forget the lessons of my experience. On the wall of my now defunct but soon to be resurrected math classroom were a few dozen inspirational quotes. Some were humorous, but most had some of level of meaning ranging from the obvious to the profound. "Never Try to Teach a Pig to Sing; It Wastes Your Time and Just Annoys the Pig." I do not know the author. Students loved that one. When Thomas Edison was asked how it felt to fail over 2,000 times before he finally succeeded in inventing the electric light bulb, he reportedly replied, "I never failed once. It was just a 2,000 step process." That, for me, says everything that needs to be said about learning and about teaching in a nutshell. A full chapter could be written about this quote. A statement so powerful, so clear, that it goes to the heart of learning and teaching. If only teachers and students could read it every day and internalize this lesson about the journey that each of them is part of; that they are *supposed* to make mistakes, and lots of them!

But there were four quotes that carried me through PTSD and then benzodiazepine addiction and withdrawal. Two that helped me gain perspective on a daily basis were in the front of my soon to be new classroom .

"I cried when I had no shoes until I met a man with no feet." This was a gentle reminder to me that no matter how bad I thought I had it, someone else was suffering more than me. Even more than that, maybe neither I nor the other man had any business complaining. After all, we are who we are, we have what we have, and we live life. Some people on this earth born without legs or arms, or born blind or deaf, are far happier than their "normal" brethren. So I read this quote and kicked myself in the pants whenever I could.

I read somewhere a statement that I can only paraphrase. The next time you start to whine or complain, remember that there are literally billions of human beings who would gladly take your burdens and swap places with you. In fact, there really ARE billions of people who would have traded places with me, even at the height of my suffering. That really caused me to think. What must their lives be like?

During the height of my two different illnesses, one a brain injury and one an addiction to a prescription medication, I tried very hard to focus on learning all that I could from the experience. For I do believe that "we can learn more from 10 days of adversity than 10 years of contentment". Putting my energy here, on learning as much as I could from the circumstances of my life, helped me immensely as I struggled not to be overly self-involved. That is an enormous challenge in benzo withdrawal, as the drug forces you to engage in countless hours of mindless self-examination and doomsday prognoses. But then one day in the midst of the benzo portion of my journey, soon to be told, I went to my little Episcopalian Church only 1.5 miles from my country home. I didn't go very often for months on end for reasons that are now obvious.

Father Brian McHugh, our Vicar, Priest, and Friend, provided a thoughtful, intelligent, funny, whimsical, often truly brilliant sermon. I came to look forward to this part of the service with a sense of anticipation. Even though, during my illness, portions of the service were extremely difficult both physically and psychologically, I was always just plain happy to know that the sermon was next. On one particular Sunday morning, Fr. Brian told a story about his days as a young Monk in a Seminary on the Hudson River. His mentor, an older Monk, was on his deathbed. Father Brian said to him, "I am so sad, not only because you are dying, but because you've had such a hard life". The dying Monk had lost many friends and family members before him, and had also suffered greatly with illnesses. He looked at Fr. Brian and said, "Brian, haven't you figured this out yet? Don't you understand that we're *supposed* to have great difficulties in our lives, that life isn't *supposed* to be easy?" There was more that followed, but that's all I needed. Everything came together. It was, for me, truly an epiphany. Our lives aren't supposed to be easy! It's okay to suffer! And when those hard times call our name, we have the best opportunity of all to learn. *We're supposed to struggle so that we can learn!* Truly learn. We can then carry that learning into the "well" stages of our lives! More than that, when tough times arrive again, *and they will*, we have a deeper reservoir from which to gain perspective and move forward, hopefully learning even more. To struggle is to grow. To suffer is to learn. All we have to do is pay attention to the lessons that are there, ready to be absorbed into our lives.

This sort of thinking completely changed my thinking about adversity. Throughout the rest of my journey through illness, it kept me above the water, helped me see through the darkness, but most of all, helped me think about my own needs less. Even in sickness, we can care about others.

I was so very high on life at that moment and for periods of time to this very day because of that lesson. I review this lesson frequently. It's okay when I get sick. When tragedy strikes, I know it will help me, though it will not be easy. I can turn that around, perhaps slowly, and make it an opportunity to learn. Thank goodness for that lesson, for it was one of the major players in my ability to defeat the most powerful adversary my life has seen.

159

Do what you think is best (DWYTIB).

- E. Robert Mercer

Chapter 32: If You Are Taking Poison

There are several million of you out there in America taking benzos, and millions more in other western countries. Read the list of potential symptoms in appendix A, and then read the list of benzos in chapter 1 carefully. If you see your medication there, you are on the edge of the bizarre, unforgiving, world of benzo addiction and withdrawal. Period. What do you do? Well, if my experience hasn't convinced you, I don't know what will. But the longer you wait, the worse things will likely be. Sure, there is always a teeny, tiny chance that you aren't addicted. But if you have any sense left in you at all, you will begin a slow taper and GET OFF. Remember, my experience is in the middle. About half of the people I have encountered in the benzo world had or are having a more difficult path and about half, a kinder path. DO NOT just stop cold turkey. You may be putting your life in jeopardy. DO NOT just stop cold turkey. If you don't suffer seizures or die, you may well be setting the stage for a long and hellish road. DO a slow taper.

There is a high probability that, sooner or later, the benzo beast will creep up on you. The longer you wait, the more terrible things will likely be. Don't wait. Resolve to get off now. Also, while is some correlation between the level of withdrawal symptoms and both the dosage and duration of benzo administration, there are so many exceptions due to individual physiology and psychology that there is no way to accurately predict what will happen during your taper. A slow, valium taper is the best way to minimize symptoms.

But if you continue to play the waiting game, you are playing with fire. Tolerance withdrawal is equivalent to my experience multiplied by some factor of ten. If you begin to experience symptoms during your regular dosing, it is not a good thing. Then, if you decide simply to increase your dosage, all you are doing is delaying the pain of withdrawal to a day when it is much worse. Get off now. NOW. Slowly. Regain a healthy life free from the ravages of these horrible drugs. Read the Dr. Heather Ashton withdrawal guidelines. It's available online. Read The Benzo Book, by Jack Hobson-Dupont. Get off. DO NOT stop cold turkey. It can kill you.

Above all, recognize that you have the power and the strength to get off these drugs. Everyone's taper is different, but the alternative to getting off NOW slowly, is bad, very, very bad. Waiting simply delays the inevitable, and the inevitable becomes worse over time.

Speak to your doctor about this. But remember that your doctor, frankly, may not have a clue. No one can possibly legitimately lay claim to knowing more about this issue than Dr. Heather Ashton. Also, go to benzo.org.uk and join the most recent version of the forum, Benzo Island. These people have hands-on experience, and you will have the benefit of the experience and wisdom of many other benzo experiencers.

And there is one more critical thing to remember. Very commonly, after a period of time, these drugs CAUSE the very symptoms that they were initially helping. This is critical. Many of you believe that you needed to take more benzos after a period of 6 months or even years because your symptoms were suddenly getting worse. It is far more likely that addiction had set in and the drugs were now your enemy, paradoxically *causing the initial symptoms or even new ones to appear.* Get off NOW, slowly.

It doesn't seem fair, but many are faced with an unpleasant choice:

1. Begin to taper now, following the guidelines of Dr. Ashton, and potentially deal with withdrawal symptoms that are unpleasant, and then win your freedom.
2. Wait for another day in the future, when the withdrawal will likely be far more difficult.

The pugilistic analogy that comes to mind is, would you prefer a left jab to the head or a right cross?

If you have never tried to stop taking benzos, there is a much better chance that your taper will be on the kind side. Most of the people at benzo.org.uk come there after an unsuccessful attempt to do a direct taper from their benzo, without the benefit of a slow, valium taper. Or, they have tried the cold turkey approach and survived, only to be beset by powerful symptoms so strong that they had no choice but to reinstate.

Do the best thing you can do for yourself. Find a doctor who will support your cross to valium and a slow, methodical taper thereafter. Join the benzo.org.uk forum or any forum of your choice. Get off these drugs. There is substantial research that indicates that the initial effects of the drugs do not last and that they are likely not helping anymore, and have turned on you.

Do not allow the pharmaceutical companies to latch onto you and keep you addicted.

Take action. Consult your doctor. If you have to, find one that will support you. Then begin your journey to benzo freedom.

And remember: YOU CAN DO IT.

Quote: Et Tu, Brute?

- William Shakespeare

Chapter 33: Torture in Our Nursing Homes

Our nursing homes are filled with mothers, fathers, grandmothers and grandfathers who have become hopelessly addicted to a classification of drugs known as benzodiazepines. You have read that correctly...ADDICTED. What's more, the symptoms of this addiction are simply horrific. And our loved ones are simply too old to withstand the attempt to withdraw from these drugs. As I indicated in the prologue, several heroin addicts have told me unequivocally, independently of one another, that detox and withdrawal from heroin is like a walk in the park compared to withdrawal from benzos.

Prescribed quickly and widely, sometimes with what seems like reasonable justification, many nursing home patients are actually being medically abused, in the humble opinion of this writer. Wandering Alzheimer's patients, for example, are easy to keep safe with "only" 1 milligram of Ativan, three times a day. This dosage initially sedates them sufficiently so that they can go nowhere. One milligram of Ativan and 10 mg. of Valium are approximately equivalent doses of two different but closely related benzos. Ten milligrams of Valium sends most non-medicated adults into a drug-induced sleep within minutes.

But there can be an enormous cost associated with this initially seemingly reasonable decision. Once addicted, a rising tide of horrible symptoms can set in, requiring an increase in dosage, which temporarily relieves symptoms. This cycle can escalate, with additional drugs prescribed to counteract "adverse side effects" until the elderly patient becomes an apparent zombie, staring into space, unmoving, the victim of a medically prescribed drug cocktail that produces symptoms above and beyond normal aging problems. Family and staff all agree that it is sad to see our loved ones age in this manner. But this is wrong; very, very wrong. They are not suffering from normal aging. No, they are suffering the effects of powerful tranquilizers that leave them drugged, lost in a world unreal beyond our understanding. Do you wonder why so many of these patients present an underlying anxiety? Do you wonder why so many of them present underlying fears? Now you have part of the answer. It is very disturbing to learn this, but it is the truth, in my humble opinion. Below is a brief excerpt from Dr. Heather Ashton's publication, Benzodiazepines: How They Work and How to Withdraw. Again, Ashton is widely considered one of the world's preeminent experts on benzodiazepines.

> **Adverse effects in the elderly.** Older people are more sensitive than younger people to the central nervous system depressant effects of benzodiazepines. Benzodiazepines can cause confusion, night wandering, amnesia, ataxia (loss of balance), hangover effects and "pseudodementia" (sometimes wrongly attributed to Alzheimer's disease) in the elderly and should be avoided wherever possible. Increased sensitivity to benzodiazepines in older people is partly because they metabolise drugs less efficiently than younger people, so that drug effects last longer and drug accumulation readily occurs with regular use. However, even at the same blood concentration, the depressant effects of benzodiazepines are greater in the elderly, possibly because they have fewer brain cells and less reserve brain capacity than younger people.
> For these reasons, it is generally advised that, if benzodiazepines are used in the elderly, dosage should be

half that recommended for adults, and use (as for adults) should be short-term (2 weeks) only.

Confusion, night wandering, amnesia, ataxia and pseudodementia, sometimes wrongly attributed to Alzheimer's! I wonder how many of loved ones are incorrectly diagnosed with Alzheimer's after beginning a course of benzos. Add to this the symptoms of benzo addiction, all caused, not by the aging process, but by one of the most if not the most commonly distributed drugs, by classification, at nursing homes across America. If this were happening to you, would you be frightened? One wonders where the outrage is. I am hopeful that it is locked within the walls of ignorance, ready to step forward boldly once knowledge sheds the light of day upon it. I pray to God that if I should ever find myself in a nursing home, there is a standing order: no benzos! I prefer lethal injection, please. The troubling truth is that our nursing homes are in such a terrible situation, so understaffed and under-scrutinized that benzos are sometimes distributed to the elderly just to keep them calm, sedated, easy to care for. How often does this happen? No one knows. But the question remains: What in God's name are we doing to loved ones?

All too often, our elderly are given benzodiazepines to simplify the lives of their caretakers. In return for this increased ease of care, our parents and grandparents are being turned into addicts. Numerous studies suggest that use of benzodiazepines may result in an increased incidence of falls, the very thing that may be identified as the reason for starting benzos (risk of falling).

The next time you wander through the hallways of a nursing home, count the number of souls you see staring into space. Look at their eyes. Do you really think that all or most of them have aged this way naturally? Think again. Many of them are trapped inside bodies that have been needlessly poisoned by benzodiazepines. For them, there is no way back. They are too frail to withdraw, unless they are among the lucky ones who are not addicted. Many will end their lives addicted to poisons that the medical profession has chosen to give them.

And read one more time the final recommendation by Ashton regarding benzodiazepines and our elderly.

For these reasons, it is generally advised that, if benzodiazepines are used in the elderly, dosage should be half that recommended for adults, and use (as for adults) should be short-term (2 weeks) only.

Ashton's recommendation is ***two weeks maximum*** for our elderly! This simply does not happen, unless a family member is amongst the few who happens to know something about this generally miserable class of medications. The truth is, once a nursing home patient has been placed on a benzodiazepine, it is likely to be with them until death, a death that can well find the patient, a loved one, drugged beyond the point of decency, experiencing terrible symptoms all the while.

And so, this notion that we send our parents, grandparents, and sometimes a spouse to a nursing home so that they can be "cared" for has a different edge now. Certainly, there is a great deal of caring in these places from special people. Some elderly care workers are truly special people, who have a loving touch in all they do. This chapter is not a carpet indictment of these workers. As in all occupations, there is a vast assortment of skills and attitudes within the ranks of nursing home employees. In my heart, I believe most of them are good people.

This is mostly about ignorance of the facts, a lack of understanding of the true effect of these drugs when misused. And make no mistake about it, they are misused. It is often easier to assign a drug to a patient than to find other ways to deal with behavior.

How can any nurse, doctor or aide, knowing what benzos are really like, knowing the true effect that they can have on an elderly patient, push forward with a long term administration? It is my hope that after reading this book, benzodiazepine administration in nursing homes will experience a precipitous drop. Anyone in the medical profession, including those in nursing homes, who reads this book surely will reconsider their actions.

There are a small number of physicians, nurses and aides who ARE aware of this and who DO use different judgment. Thank God for these people. But right now, knowledge of the addictive qualities and difficulty of withdrawal is NOT common knowledge, and it ought to be. It's up to those of us who have suffered through the ordeal of benzodiazepine withdrawal to spread the word, and now it's up to you, too.

Appendix A

Symptom List (Benzo.org.uk)

1. ACUTE:

- aggression
- anxiety
- agoraphobia
- apathy
- ataxia
- breathlessness
- chest discomfort and tightness
- choking
- constipation
- convulsions (muscle usually)
- dental pain
- depersonalisation
- depression
- derealisation
- diarrhoea
- distortion of body image, misperceptions
- dry, itchy skin
- "electric shock" feelings throughout the body
- dysphoria
- excitability
- fasciculations
- flushing
- formications
- head sensations
- heart palpitations
- hyperacusis
- hypersensitivity to stimuli
- hyperosmia (sensitive sense of smell)
- hyperpyrexia (overheating)
- hyperventilation (overbreathing)
- insomnia

- intrusive thoughts
- irrational rage
- irritability
- jumpiness
- metallic taste
- nausea
- nightmares
- obsessions
- panic attacks
- perceptual disturbances and distortions
- photosensitivity
- psychotic symptoms (usually transient and
  confined to rapid withdrawal)
- restlessness
- seizures (on abrupt discontinuation)
- sensory disruption
- scalp burning
- sore tongue
- sweating, night sweats
- tinnitus
- tremor
- vomiting
- weakness, "jelly legs"
- weight gain
- weight loss (this may be quite rapid)

Cold Turkey
Symptoms usually confined to 'cold turkey' or rapid
withdrawal from high doses of benzodiazepines:

- confusion
- delirium
- fits
- hallucinations
- psychotic symptoms
- seizures

2. PROTRACTED:

- abnormal muscle tone
- anxiety
- aching joints
- ataxia
- allergic reactions
- back pain
- blepharospasm (eye twitching)
- breast pain
- apathy
- constipation (often alternating with diarrhoea)
- cravings
- dehydration
- dental pain
- depersonalisation
- depression
- derealisation
- diarrhoea (often alternating with constipation)
- dry, tickly cough
- dysphagia
- fluctuations in blood pressure
- "electric shock" feelings throughout the body
- fasciculations
- formication (sensation of bugs crawling over skin)
- gait disturbance (the ground seems to move underfoot)
- gastritis
- glassy eyes
- hair loss
- heartburn
- heart palpitations
- heavy flu-like symptoms
- hyperacusis
- hyperaesthesia (sensitivity to stimuli)
- hyperosmia
- insomnia
- iris colour changes
- kakosmia

- joint pains
- leukonychea (whitening of nails)
- libidinal changes
- malabsorption
- menstrual irregularity
- muscular cramps
- muscular rigidity
- muscular spasms
- muscular (and bone) weakness
- myoclonic convulsions (muscle/nerve spasms)
- nausea
- neurological problems (topical nerve anaesthesia)
- nose bleeds
- oedema (especially of ankles and face)
- oesophagitis
- paraesthesiae (numbing, burning and tingling; pins and needles)
- poor concentration
- poor short-term memory
- perspiring, night sweats
- severe headaches
- sinusitis
- skin insensitivity
- sore, itchy eyes
- spine (burning sensation)
- stomach cramps
- thirst
- thrush-like symptoms
- tremor
- tinnitus (ear buzzing, popping, ringing, hissing)
- tiny pupils
- urinary problems (bladder either 'all on' or 'all off')
- vertigo
- visual disturbances (blurred, double, vivid)
- vomiting
- water retention

3. PARADOXICAL:

- acute hyperexcited state
- agitation
- aggressive behaviour
- anxiety
- breathlessness
- excitability
- fear
- hallucinations
- hostility
- hyperactivity
- increased muscle spasticity
- irrational rage
- insomnia
- nervousness
- nightmares, vivid dreams
- phobias
- rage
- restlessness
- restless legs, arms
- sleep disturbances
- tension
- tremor
- panic attacks

4. TOLERANCE EFFECTS (including toxicity):

- anxiety
- apnea (night)
- breathlessness
- dyspnea (breathing problems)
- fibrositis
- fatigue
- gait disturbance
- impotence
- leaden heaviness
- lethargy
- libido disturbances
- loss of self-confidence
- menstrual irregularity

- neurological problems
- panic attacks
- phobias
- severe muscle rigidity
- short-term memory impairment
- vasovagal attacks
- vertigo

5. SIDE EFFECTS:

- abnormal behaviour or false beliefs
- aches and pains (muscle tension)
- aggressiveness
- agitation
- agoraphobia and claustrophobia
- anger
- anti-social behaviour
- apathy
- ataxia
- blood disorders (resulting in severe tiredness
  and possible infections)
- blurred vision
- bradycardia (slow heartbeat/pulse)
- breast enlargement
- changes in appetite
- changes in libido
- changes in salivation
- chemical sensitivities, allergies
- cognitive impairment
- confusion
- daytime drowsiness
- depression
- diarrhoea and constipation
- diplopia
- dizziness
- dry, itchy skin
- dysarthria
- dysphoria
- emotional blunting
- exhaustion

- fatigue
- feeling afraid
- feeling unreal
- feelings of anger and anxiety
- flu-like symptoms
- hair loss
- hallucinations
- headaches
- hypotension
- IBS (Irritable Bowel Syndrome)
- inability to pass urine/holding of urine in the bladder
- impairment of motor co-ordination
- incontinence
- insomnia
- irritability
- jaundice
- jaw pains
- lack of concentration
- lack of confidence
- lethargy
- many people wonder why they have changed from being happy
  and outgoing, to being over-anxious and unconfident
- memory loss or forgetfulness
- mild hypertension
- muscle weakness, spasticity, cramps, abnormal tone
- nausea
- nightmares
- numbed emotions
- oedema
- panic attacks
- personality changes
- poor muscle control
- problems with vision
- psychomotor impairment
- rashes
- reduced alertness
- reduced blood pressure

- restlessness
- shivering
- skin problems, rashes
- sleep problems
- slurred speech
- stomach and bowel problems
- stomach upsets
- suicidal behaviour
- thyroid disturbances
- tolerance
- tremor
- urinary retention
- vertigo
- violence
- water retention
- weight gain
- xeroderma (dry skin)

6. CATEGORIES OF SYMPTOMS:

CARDIOVASCULAR:

Fluctuations in blood pressure
Mild hypertension
Shivering, feelings of extreme cold or hot
Heart palpitations

DERMATOLOGICAL:

Allergic reactions
Chemical sensitivities
Dry, itchy skin
Dry throat, sore tongue, and thrush
Formications (sensation of crawling on skin)
Glassy eyes
Hair loss
Leukonychea (whitening of nails)
Nosebleeds
Oedema
Paraesthesiae (numbness, tingling)

Perspiring, night sweats
Rashes, blotches

GASTROINTESTINAL:

Bladder incontinence
Constipation (sometimes alternating with diarrhoea)
Diarrhoea
Dyspepsia (indigestion)
Gastritis
Heartburn
Nausea
Oesophagitis
Stomach cramps

GENITOURINARY:

Impotence
Libido disturbances
Menstrual irregularities
urinary problems (continence or incontinence)
Encopressia (faecal incontinence)

MUSCULOSKELETAL:

Aching joints
Blepharospasm (eye twitches)
Formication (sensations of bugs crawling on skin)
Gait disturbance
Jaw, tooth, neck and shoulder pain
Muscle wasting
Muscle spasms
Rapid weight loss
Severe headaches
Severe muscle rigidity
Tremor or feeling of inner vibration
Vertigo

NEUROLOGICAL:

Blurred vision, seeing spots, flashes, vivid
vision
Bruxism (teeth grinding)
Dysphagia (difficulty eating or swallowing)
Electric shock feelings
Fatigue, leaden heaviness
Hypersensitivity to light, sound, and other
stimuli
Neurological problems (e.g. topical
anaesthesia)
Severe muscle rigidity
Speech difficulty
Thirst
Tinnitus (ear buzzing, popping, ringing,
hissing)
Tiny pupils
Tremor

PARADOXICAL:

Agitation
Aggressive behaviour anxiety
Breathlessness
Excitability
Fear
Hostility
Hyperactivity
Irrational rage
Insomnia
Nervousness
Nightmares, vivid dreams
Phobias
Restlessness

PSYCHIATRIC:

Apathy
Anxiety

Delirium
Depersonalisation
Depression
Derealisation
Distortions or hallucinations
Dysphoria (inability to feel pleasure or happiness)
Fear
Hyperventilation
Hyperreflexia ('jumpiness')
Hypnologic hallucinations sleepwalking)
Lack of concentration
Nightmares
Obsessions
Paranoia
Phobias (hydrophobia, agoraphobia, monophobia, acrophobia, anthropophobia and others)
Rapid mood changes
Suicidal thoughts
Short-term memory impairment

RESPIRATORY:

Breathlessness
Choking
Dry, tickly cough
Dyspnea (breathing difficulty)
Hyperventilation (overbreathing)
Inability to draw satisfying breath
Night apnea
Sinusitis

These lists are pretty comprehensive and include symptoms reported by members of the Benzo Group. It is mercifully unlikely that any one person will experience all the symptoms recorded here. They are given purely for reference purposes.

Note: It is difficult to determine exactly which symptoms are acute and which are protracted. Everyone's experience is clearly different.

Ray Nimmo and others from the Benzo Group · July 2000.

Common symptoms of PTSD and Complex PTSD

- hypervigilance (feels like but is *not* paranoia)
- exaggerated startle response
- irritability
- sudden angry or violent outbursts
- flashbacks, nightmares, intrusive recollections, replays, violent visualizations
- triggers
- sleep disturbance
- exhaustion and chronic fatigue
- reactive depression
- guilt
- feelings of detachment
- avoidance behaviours
- nervousness, anxiety
- phobias about specific daily routines, events or objects
- irrational or impulsive behaviour
- loss of interest
- loss of ambition
- anhedonia (inability to feel joy and pleasure)
- poor concentration
- impaired memory
- joint pains, muscle pains
- emotional numbness
- physical numbness
- low self-esteem
- an overwhelming sense of injustice and a strong desire to do something about it

Appendix C

Differences between mental illness and psychiatric injury
(source: an undetermined website)

Paranoia	Hypervigilance
• paranoia is a form of mental *illness*; the cause is thought to be internal, e.g. a minor variation in the balance of brain chemistry	• is a response to an external event (violence, accident, disaster, violation, intrusion, bullying, etc) and therefore an *injury*
• paranoia tends to endure and to not get better of its own accord	• wears off (gets better), albeit slowly, when the person is out of and away from the situation which was the cause
• the paranoiac will not admit to feeling paranoid, as they cannot see their paranoia	• the hypervigilant person is acutely aware of their hypervigilance, and will easily articulate their fear, albeit using the incorrect but popularised word "paranoia"
• sometimes responds to drug treatment	• drugs are not viewed favourably by hypervigilant people, except in extreme

	circumstances, and then only briefly; often drugs have no effect, or can make things worse, sometimes interfering with the body's own healing process
• the paranoiac often has delusions of grandeur; the delusional aspects of paranoia feature in other forms of mental illness, such as schizophrenia	• the hypervigilant person often has a diminished sense of self-worth, sometimes dramatically so
• the paranoiac is convinced of their self-importance	• the hypervigilant person is often convinced of their worthlessness and will often deny their value to others
• paranoia is often seen in conjunction with other symptoms of mental illness, but *not* in conjunction with symptoms of PTSD	• hypervigilance is seen in conjunction with other symptoms of PTSD, but *not* in conjunction with symptoms of mental illness
• the paranoiac is convinced of their plausibility	• the hypervigilant person is aware of how implausible their experience sounds and often doesn't want to believe it themselves

	(disbelief and denial)
• the paranoiac feels persecuted by a person or persons unknown (eg "*they're* out to get me")	• the hypervigilant person is hypersensitized but is often aware of the inappropriateness of their heightened sensitivity, and can identify the person responsible for their psychiatric injury
• sense of persecution	• heightened sense of vulnerability to victimisation
• the sense of persecution felt by the paranoiac is a delusion, for usually no-one is out to get them	• the hypervigilant person's sense of threat is well-founded, for the serial bully *is* out to get rid of them and has often coerced others into assisting, eg through mobbing; the hypervigilant person often cannot (and refuses to) see that the serial bully is doing everything possible to get rid of them
• the paranoiac is on constant alert because they *know* someone is out to get them	• the hypervigilant person is on alert *in case* there is danger

• the paranoiac is certain of their belief and their behaviour and expects others to share that certainty	• the hypervigilant person cannot bring themselves to believe that the bully cannot and will not see the effect their behaviour is having; they cling naively to the mistaken belief that the bully will recognise their wrongdoing and apologise

Other differences between mental illness and psychiatric injury include:

Mental illness	Psychiatric injury
• the cause often cannot be identified	• the cause is easily identifiable and verifiable, but denied by those who are accountable
• the person may be incoherent or what they say doesn't make sense	• the person is often articulate but prevented from articulation by being traumatised
• the person may appear to	• the person is obsessive, especially in relation to

be obsessed	identifying the cause of their injury and both dealing with the cause and effecting their recovery
• the person is oblivious to their behaviour and the effect it has on others	• the person is in a state of acute self-awareness and aware of their state, but often unable to explain it
• the depression is a clinical or endogenous depression	• the depression is reactive; the chemistry is different to endogenous depression
• there may be a history of depression in the family	• there is very often *no* history of depression in the individual or their family
• the person has usually exhibited mental health problems before	• often there is *no* history of mental health problems
• may respond inappropriately to the needs and concerns of others	• responds empathically to the needs and concerns of others, *despite* their own injury
• displays a certitude about themselves, their circumstances and their actions	• is often highly skeptical about their condition and circumstances and is in a state of disbelief and bewilderment which they will easily and often

	articulate
• may suffer a persecution complex	• may experience an unusually heightened sense of vulnerability to possible victimisation (ie hypervigilance)
• suicidal thoughts are the result of despair, dejection and hopelessness	• suicidal thoughts are often a logical and carefully thought-out solution or conclusion
• exhibits despair	• is driven by the anger of injustice
• often doesn't look forward to each new day	• looks forward to each new day as an opportunity to fight for justice
• is often ready to give in or admit defeat	• refuses to be beaten, refuses to give up

Appendix D (Ashton www.benzo.org.uk)

THE BENZODIAZEPINES

Potency. A large number of benzodiazepines are available (Table 1). There are major differences in potency between different benzodiazepines, so that equivalent doses vary as much as 20-fold. For example, 0.5 milligrams (mg) of alprazolam (Xanax) is approximately equivalent to 10mg of diazepam (Valium). Thus a person on 6mg of alprazolam daily, a dose not uncommonly prescribed in the US, is taking the equivalent of about 120mg of diazepam, a very high dose. These differences in strength have not always been fully appreciated by doctors, and some would not agree with the equivalents given here. Nevertheless, people on potent benzodiazepines such as alprazolam, Lorazepam (Ativan) or clonazepam (Klonopin) tend to be using relatively large doses. This difference in potency is important when switching from one benzodiazepine to another, for example changing to diazepam during the withdrawal, as described in the next chapter.

Speed of elimination. Benzodiazepines also differ markedly in the speed at which they are metabolised (in the liver) and eliminated from the body (in the urine) (Table 1). For example, the "half-life" (time taken for the blood concentration to fall to half its initial value after a single dose) for triazolam (Halcion) is only 2-5 hours, while the half-life of diazepam is 20-100 hours, and that of an active metabolite of diazepam (desmethyldiazepam) is 36-200 hours. This means that half the active products of diazepam are still in the bloodstream up to 200 hours after a single dose. Clearly, with repeated daily dosing accumulation occurs and high concentrations can build up in the body (mainly in fatty tissues). As Table 1 shows, there is a considerable variation between individuals in the rate at which they metabolise benzodiazepines.

Table 1. BENZODIAZEPINES AND SIMILAR DRUGS[5]

Benzodiazepines[5]	Half-life (hrs)[1] [active metabolite]	Market Aim[2]	Approximately Equivalent Oral dosages (mg)[3]
Alprazolam (Xanax)	6-12	a	0.5
Bromazepam (Lexotan, Lexomil)	10-20	a	5-6
Chlordiazepoxide (Librium)	5-30 [36-200]	a	25
Clobazam (Frisium)	12-60	a,e	20
Clonazepam (Klonopin, Rivotril)	18-50	a,e	0.5
Clorazepate (Tranxene)	[36-200]	a	15
Diazepam (Valium)	20-100 [36-200]	a	10
Estazolam (ProSom)	10-24	h	1-2
Flunitrazepam (Rohypnol)	18-26 [36-200]	h	1
Flurazepam (Dalmane)	[40-250]	h	15-30
Halazepam (Paxipam)	[30-100]	a	20
Ketazolam (Anxon)	2	a	15-30
Loprazolam (Dormonoct)	6-12	h	1-2
Lorazepam (Ativan)	10-20	a	1
Lormetazepam (Noctamid)	10-12	h	1-2
Medazepam (Nobrium)	36-200	a	10
Nitrazepam (Mogadon)	15-38	h	10
Nordazepam (Nordaz, Calmday)	36-200	a	10

Oxazepam (Serax, Serenid, Serepax)	4-15	a	20
Prazepam (Centrax)	[36-200]	a	10-20
Quazepam (Doral)	25-100	h	20
Temazepam (Restoril, Normison, Euhypnos)	8-22	h	20
Triazolam (Halcion)	2	h	0.5
Non-benzodiazepines with similar effects[4,5]			
Zaleplon (Sonata)	2	h	20
Zolpidem (Ambien, Stilnoct)	2	h	20
Zopiclone (Zimovane, Imovane)	5-6	h	15

1. Half-life: time taken for blood concentration to fall to half its peak value after a single dose. Half-life of active metabolite shown in square brackets. This time may vary considerably between individuals.
2. Market aim: although all benzodiazepines have similar actions, they are usually marketed as anxiolytics (a), hypnotics (h) or anticonvulsants (e).
3. These equivalents do not agree with those used by some authors. They are firmly based on clinical experience but may vary between individuals.
4. These drugs are chemically different from benzodiazepines but have the same effects on the body and act by the same mechanisms.
5. All these drugs are recommended for short-term use only (2-4 weeks maximum).

Duration of effects. The speed of elimination of a benzodiazepine is obviously important in determining the duration of its effects. However, the duration of apparent action is usually

189

considerably less than the half-life. With most benzodiazepines, noticeable effects usually wear off within a few hours. Nevertheless the drugs, as long as they are present, continue to exert subtle effects within the body. These effects may become apparent during continued use or may appear as withdrawal symptoms when dosage is reduced or the drug is stopped.

Therapeutic actions of benzodiazepines.

Regardless of their potency, speed of elimination or duration of effects, the actions in the body are virtually the same for all benzodiazepines. This is true whether they are marketed as anxiolytics, hypnotics or anti-convulsants (Table 1). All benzodiazepines exert five major effects which are used therapeutically: anxiolytic, hypnotic, muscle relaxant, anticonvulsant and amnesic (impairment of memory) (Table 2).

Table 2. THERAPEUTIC ACTIONS OF BENZODIAZEPINES (IN SHORT-TERM USE)

Action	Clinical Use
Anxiolytic - relief of anxiety	- Anxiety and panic disorders, phobias
Hypnotic - promotion of sleep	- Insomnia
Myorelaxant - muscle relaxation	- Muscle spasms, spastic disorders
Anticonvulsant - stop fits, convulsions	- Fits due to drug poisoning, some forms of epilepsy
Amnesia - impair short-term memory	- Premedication for operations, sedation for minor surgical procedures

Other clinical uses, utilising combined effects:

• Alcohol detoxification

• Acute psychosis with hyperexcitability and aggressiveness

These actions, exerted by different benzodiazepines in slightly varying degrees, confer on the drugs some useful medicinal properties. Few drugs can compete with them in efficacy, rapid onset of action and low acute toxicity. In short-term use, benzodiazepines can be valuable, sometimes even life-saving, across a wide range of clinical conditions as shown in Table 2. Nearly all the disadvantages of benzodiazepines result from long-term use (regular use for more than a few weeks). The UK Committee on Safety of Medicines in 1988 recommended that benzodiazepines should in general be reserved for short-term use (2-4 weeks only).

Mechanisms of action. Anyone struggling to get off their benzodiazepines will be aware that the drugs have profound effects on the mind and body apart from the therapeutic actions. Directly or indirectly, benzodiazepines in fact influence almost every aspect of brain function. For those interested to know how and why, a short explanation follows of the mechanisms through which benzodiazepines are able to exert such widespread effects.

All benzodiazepines act by enhancing the actions of a natural brain chemical, GABA (gamma-aminobutyric acid). GABA is a neurotransmitter, an agent which transmits messages from one brain cell (neuron) to another. The message that GABA transmits is an inhibitory one: it tells the neurons that it contacts to slow down or stop firing. Since about 40% of the millions of neurons all over the brain respond to GABA, this means that GABA has a general quietening influence on the brain: it is in some ways the body's natural hypnotic and tranquilliser. This natural action of GABA is augmented by benzodiazepines which thus exert an extra (often excessive) inhibitory influence on neurons

Appendix E: The Author's Tapering Schedule

Date	Cut (in Mg.)	Days between cuts/cross s	Dosage (in Mg.)	Percent of total
11/9/03		--	2.4 A/0 V	
11/16/03		7	2.0 A/4 V	
11/22/03		6	1.6 A/8 V	
11/26/03		4	1.2 A/12 V	
11/29/03		3	.8 A/16 V	
12/2/03		3	.4 A/20 V	
12/05/03	---	--	24 V	---
12/12/03	2	--	22	8%
12/24/03	2	12	20	9%
1/4/04	2	11	18	10%
1/15/04	2	11	16	11%
1/29/04	1	14	15	6.3%
2/11/04	1	13	14	6.7%
2/22/04	1	11	13	7.2%
3/2/04	.5	8	12.5	3.8%
3/8/04	.5	7	12	4%
3/15/04	.5	7	11.5	4.2%
3/22/04	.5	7	11	4.3%
3/29/04	.5	7	10.5	4.5%
4/5/04	.5	7	10	4.8%

4/12/04	.5	7	9.5	5%
4/19/04	.5	7	9	5.3%
4/26/04	.5	7	8.5	5.6%
5/3/04	.5	7	8	5.9%
5/10/04	.5	7	7.5	6.3%
5/17/04	.5	7	7	6.7%
5/26/04	.5	9	6.5	7.1%
6/6/04	.5	11	6	7.6%
6/15/05	.5	9	5.5	8.3%
6/25/04	.5	10	5	9%
7/4/04	.5	9	4.5	10%
7/14/04	.5	10	4	11.1%
7/24/04	.5	10	3.5	12.5%
8/3/04	.5	10	3	14.3%
8/13/04	.5	10	2.5	16.7%
8/23/04	.5	10	2	20%
9/2/04	.5	10	1.5	25%
9/12/04	.5	10	1	33.3%
9/22/04	.5	10	.5	50%
10/2/04	.5	10	0	100%

Total time taken to taper, including crossover to diazepam: 11 months.

Appendix F

SUGGESTED REFERENCES

Following is a selection of articles and papers from the more than 200 that Heather Ashton, M.D. has written. These articles can be found at www.benzo.org.uk or at www.benzosupport.org.

- Overprescribing of Benzodiazepines: Problems and Resolutions, 3rd Annual Benzodiazepine Conference in Bangor, Maine, October 11, 2005.
- History of Benzodiazepines: What the Textbooks May Not Tell You, 3rd Annual Benzodiazepine Conference in Bangor, Maine, October 12, 2005.
- Protracted Withdrawal Symptoms from Benzodiazepines, 2004.
- Benzodiazepines: How they Work & How to Withdraw (The Ashton Manual), 2002.
- Benzodiazepine Abuse, 2002.
- Benzodiazepines & Older People, March, 2002. [Dansk version]
- A View from the Shoulders of Giants. A Review of David Healy's "The Psychopharmacologists III", September 2001.
- "Chemical Imbalance", August 28, 2001.
- Benzodiazepine Equivalence Table, June 2001.
- Reasons for a diazepam (Valium) taper, April 2001.

- Guidelines for Withdrawal of Antidepressant Drugs, January 2001.
- SSRIs, Drug Withdrawal and Abuse: Problem or Treatment? C. Heather Ashton and Allan H. Young, 1999.
- Benzodiazepine Dependency, 1997.
- Long-Term Effects of Benzodiazepine Usage: Research Proposals, 1995-96.
- Protracted Withdrawal From Benzodiazepines: The Post-Withdrawal Syndrome, March 1995. [Dansk version]
- Toxicity and Adverse Consequences of Benzodiazepine Use, March 1995.
- The Treatment of Benzodiazepine Dependence, 1994.
- Guidelines for the Rational Use of Benzodiazepines, When and What to Use, 1994.
- Protracted Withdrawal Syndromes from Benzodiazepines, 1991.
- Helping patients come off benzodiazepines, The Pulse, July 22, 1989.
- Risks of dependence on benzodiazepine drugs: a major problem of long term treatment, January 1989.
- A problem with Lorazepam? 1988.
- Doctors turn to more addictive short-acting benzodiazepines, Druglink 1988.
- Benzodiazepine Withdrawal: Outcome in 50 Patients, 1987.
- Adverse Effects of Prolonged Benzodiazepine Use, June, 1986.
- Benzodiazepine Withdrawal. Introductory Message at Carol Packer's benzodiazepine.org web site.

Additional Articles:

Review of Behavioral Effects of Benzodiazepines By Dr Peter Breggin (can be found at www.benzosupport.org under "Information" tab) NOTE: Dr. Breggin's background includes a teaching fellowship at Harvard Medical School, a two-year appointment to the National Institute of Mental Health (NIMH), and a faculty appointment to the Johns Hopkins University Department of Counseling.

Benzodiazepine Warning to Doctors (also at www.benzosupport.org)

Extracts From Articles in Medical Publications on the Physical, Psychological and Social Decline of Long Term Benzodiazepine Users (www.benzosupport.org under Dr. Reg Peart)

The Benzodiazepines Toxicity, Cognitive Impairment, Long-Term Damage & The Post Withdrawal Syndrome (also under Dr. Reg Peart at above website)

"Review of Behavioral Effects of Benzodiazepines with an Appendix on Drawing Scientific Conclusions from the FDA's Spontaneous Reporting System" by Peter Breggin, M.D. (Medwatch) (Can be found at www.breggin.com)

"Suppressing the Passion of Anxiety Overwhelm with Drugs: The Minor Tranquilizers, Including Xanax, Valium, BuSpar, Ativan, and Halcion, and the Antidepressant Anafranil" by Peter Breggin (excerpted from Toxic Psychiatry by Peter Breggin and can be found at www.breggin.com).

"Benefits and Risks of Benzodiazepines in Anxiety and Insomnia." Professor Malcolm Lader, Professor of Clinical Psychopharmacology, Institute of Psychiatry, University of London.

"Persistence of Cognitive Effects After Withdrawal from Long-Term Benzodiazepine Use: A Meta-Analysis." Barker M.J., Greenwood, K.M., Jackson M., and Crowe S.F. Arch. Clin. Neuropsychol. 2004 April.

"The Prolonged Benzodiazepine Withdrawal Syndrome: Anxiety or Hysteria?" Higgitt A., Fonagy P., Toone B., and Shine P. Acta Psychiatr Scand., Aug. 1990.

"Different GABAa Receptor Subtypes Mediate the Anxiolytic, Abuse-Related, and Motor Effects of Benzodiazepine-Like Drugs in Primates." James K. Rowlett, Donna M. Platt, Snjezana Lelas, John R. Atack, and Gerard R. Dawson.

"Basic Pharmacologic Mechanisms Involved in Benzodiazepine Tolerance and Withdrawal." A. N. Bateson. *Current Pharmaceutical Design*. 2002, 8, 5-21.

"Possible Interaction of Fluoroquinolones with the Benzodiazepine-GABAa Receptor Complex." Elizabeth Unseld, G. Ziegler,A. Gemeinhardt, U. Janssen and U. Klotz. *Br. J. Clinc. Pharmac.* 1999, 30, 63-70.

"Benzodiazepine Tolerance, Dependency and Withdrawal Syndromes, the Benzodiazepine Gamma-Amino-Butyric-Acid (GABA) Receptor Complex and Its Interactions with Fluoroquinolone Antimicrobials." Dr. J. G. McConnell, BSc, M.D., FRCP, FRCPEd.

"Microsomal Metabolismof Ciprofloxacin Generates Free Radicals." Aylin G. Urbay, Brigitte Gonthier, Denis Daveloose, Alain Favier, and Filiz Hincal. *Free Radical Biology & Medicine,* Vol. 30, No. 10.

"Down-Regulation of Benzodiazepine Binding to a5 Subunit-Containing g-Aminobutyric AcidA Receptors in Tolerant Rat Brain Indicates Particular Involvement of the Hippocampal CA1 Region 1." Ming Li, Andras Szabo, and Howard C. Rosenberg. *Journal of Pharmacology and Experimental Therapeutics.* Vol. 295, No. 2.

"A Pilot Study of the Effects of Flumazenil on Symptoms Persisting After Benzodiazepine Withdrawal." Malcolm H. Lader and Sally V. Morton. *Journal of Psychopharmacology* 6(3) (1992) 357-363.

"Sedative but Not Anxiolytic Properties of Benzodiazepines are Mediated by the GABAa Receptor a1 Subtype." R. M. McKernan, T. W. Rosahl, D. S. Reynolds, C. Sur, K. A. Wafford, J. R. Atack, S. Farrar, J. Myers, G. Cook, P. Ferris, L. Garrett, L. Bristow, G. Marshall, A. Macaulay, N. Brown, O. Howell, K. W. Moore, R. W. Carling, L. J. Street, J. L. Castro, C. I. Ragan, G. R. Dawson and P. J. Whiting. *Nature Neuroscience.* Volume 3, No. 6, June 2000.

"Chronic Benzodiazepine Treatment of Cells Expressing Recombinant GABAa Receptors Uncouples Allosteric Binding: Studies on Possible Mechanisms." Noore Ali and Richard W. Olsen. *Journal of Neurochemistry,* 2001, 79, 1100-1108.

"The Basic Biochemistry of Neuropharmacology." Cooper, Bloom & Roth. Eaton T. Fores Research Center. 2002.

"Chronic Benzodiazepine Treatment Decreases Postsynaptic GABA Sensitivity." Gallager D. W., Lakoski, J. M., Gonsalves S. F., and Rauch S. L. *Nature.* 1984 Mar. 1-7; 308 (5954): 74-7.

"A Pilot Study of the Effects of Flumazenil on Symptoms Persisting after Benzodiazepine Withdrawal." Malcolm H. Lader and Sally V. Morton. *Journal of Psychopharmacology.* 6 (3) (1992) 357-363.

"Horrifying Legacy of the "Celebrity Sedative' Marketed Without Tests." Lucy Johnston and Jonathan Calvert. *Sunday Express.* October 29, 2000.

"The Diagnosis and Management of Benzodiazepine Dependence." Heather Ashton, M.D. *Current Opinion in Psychiatry.* 2005. 249-255.

BOOKS:

ADDICTION BY PRESCRIPTION by Joan E. Gadsby.

ACCIDENTAL ADDICT by Di Porritt and Di Russell.

THE ANTIDEPRESSANT FACT BOOK: WHAT YOUR DOCTOR WON'T TELL YOU ABOUT PROZAC, ZOLOFT, PAXIL, CELEXA AND LUVOX by Peter Breggin, M.D.

THE DARK SIDE OF SLEEPING PILLS by Daniel F. Kripke, M.D.

YOUR DRUG MAY BE YOUR PROBLEM: HOW AND WHY TO STOP TAKING PSYCHIATRIC MEDICATIONS by Peter Breggin, M.D. and David Cohen, PhD.

THE RITALIN FACT BOOK: WHAT YOUR DOCTOR WON'T TELL YOU ABOUT ADHD AND STIMULANT DRUGS by Peter Breggin, M.D.

TOXIC PSYCHIATRY by Peter Breggin, M.D.

TALKING BACK TO PROZAC: WHAT DOCTORS AREN'T TELLING YOU ABOUT TODAY'S MOST CONTROVERSIAL DRUG by Peter Breggin, M.D.

PROZAC BACKLASH by Joseph Glenmullen, M.D.

THE BENZO BOOK by Jack Hobson-Dupont

BENZO BLUES by Sam Drummond, M.D.

PROZAC: PANACEA OR PANDORA? by Ann Blake Tracy, PhD.

ON-LINE SUPPORT GROUPS and/or INFORMATIONAL SITES:

www.benzo.org.uk

www.bcnc.org.uk

www.benzosupport.org

www.benzosupport.org

www.tranx.org.au (Australia).

www.benzohelp.com   (Out of Boulder, Colorado. Alison Kellagher, M.A., does private support counseling for those with benzodiazepine addiction/withdrawal).

As long as you are trying to be something other than what you actually are, your mind merely wears itself out. But if you say, "This is what I am, it is a fact that I am going to investigate, understand", then you can go beyond.

Krishnamurti (1891-1986)

Made in the USA
San Bernardino, CA
19 September 2013